Endorsements

"As a family physician, I acknowledge the importance of delivering health information in a very simple way. To get healthy does not mean to navigate a complex medical system, or to use the most recent medications as many times portrayed in the media. To be healthy consists in following practical steps as presented in this book by Dr. Dona Cooper-Dockery. I strongly encourage everybody to engage in reading this book. Hope you enjoy it, and concurrently get healthy."
　　— **Ubaldo Salazar, M.D.,** Family Practice Physician

"Dr. Cooper-Dockery has brilliantly crafted a tool that if you take the time to understand it and use for yourself, your family, and your institution, you could live smarter, longer, healthier, happier, save a bundle of money, and in the process, help secure your retirement."
　　— **Errol B. Bryce, M.D., FACP,** President, *New Steps to Health*; Adj. Asst. Professor of Medicine, UNT HSC

"If you want to live a longer, stronger, and more energetic life, then you've found the solution in this timely book, *Get Healthy for Life*. The title says it all. Take charge of your health and you will find that every other area of your life improves. The ball is in your court. Start reading and get healthy for life now."

— **Randrick Chance,** Founder of *Strategic Secrets*; pastor and lifestyle coach; #1 bestselling author of *Prayers that Move Heaven* and *Monetize Your Skills*

"My experience with the Cooper-Dockery Wellness Center began following my visit with Dr. Cooper-Dockery for an annual checkup. My physical condition was not good. I was extremely overweight, my blood pressure was high (150/110), I had shortness of breath, my knees hurt because of the excess weight and old surgeries, and I had no stamina at all. A short walk of 10 minutes was all I could muster before I had to rest. So, Dr. Cooper-Dockery suggested that I talk to the folks at her wellness clinic. At first, I was skeptical and reluctant, but after I met with the members of the staff, I decided to join the wellness center.

During the following 5½ months, the staff at the center helped, encouraged, and inspired me in my journey. What they helped me accomplish was nothing short of a miracle. At the end of the 5½ months, I had lost 60 pounds, my blood pressure was perfectly normal (120/70), and I had no shortness of breath at all. I was walking for over an hour each day for at least 5 days per week and on most weeks 6 days, for a total of about 4 miles. Best of all, I had no pain in my knees and legs during or after my walks.

"As I have said, the transformation was miraculous. I will be forever grateful to the group of professionals at the Cooper-Dockery Wellness Center who helped and inspired me in my journey to a healthier life. I highly recommend the center to anyone who needs help reaching a healthier lifestyle. With one's dedication and commitment, the wonderful staff at the Cooper-Dockery Wellness Center is ready to help anyone achieve their goal."

— Ronald B. Davy, Ph.D., Veterinary Entomology

"*Get Healthy for Life* gives great insights into what God intended for us to be and that is, to prosper and be in good health. Here's your ticket to having life and life more abundantly. Dr. Dona Cooper-Dockery shows us that it can start right here and now. She brings a lifelong commitment and enthusiasm with a practical approach to getting healthy and staying healthy. I know the book will be a great blessing to all who read its pages."

— Encile Brown, Ph.D.,
Senior Pastor, Mission Hope SDA Church

"After reading Dr. Cooper-Dockery's *Get Healthy for Life* I came to two incredible conclusions: The medical establishment and the drug companies will hate it and the reader will love it. The book empowers people to live a longer and healthier life and teaches individuals how to lead a lifestyle that can in most cases free them from prescription medications and dangerous and expensive medical procedures. The application of the health principles stated in this book can prevent and reverse many diseases, helping everybody to protect their most valuable assets: their physical and mental health."

— Silmar Cristo, M.D.,
Founder and Director, *Health 4D International*

"The Nine Secret Pillars of Health that Dr. Dona Cooper-Dockery has sketched in her riveting book, *Get Healthy For Life* will navigate you on how to better treat our modern-day diseases with simple and yet effective ways. Not only it uplifts you but also compels you to heed these laws of health. Its combination of health principles with spiritual insights is truly inspiring."

– Ferdinand O. Regalado, Ph.D.,
Senior pastor, *Edinburg SDA Church*

GET HEALTHY FOR LIFE

THE 9 SECRET PILLARS TO LIVE A LONGER, STRONGER, AND ENERGETIC LIFE

DONA COOPER-DOCKERY, M.D.

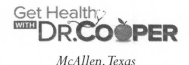

McAllen, Texas

Get Healthy with Dr. Cooper™
3604 N. McColl Road
McAllen, TX 78501
www.Gethealthywithdrcooper.tv

Medical Disclaimer:
Every effort has been made to ensure that the information contained in this book is complete and accurate. However, the ideas, procedures, and suggestions contained herein are not intended as a substitute for consulting with your physician. This book is intended to educate, inspire, and empower you to make lifestyle changes that will propel to a healthier, happier, and more fulfilled life. You should use information received in this book wisely, always consult with your primary healthcare provider if you have questions or concerns. The information received in this book should be used to supplement not to replace medical advice from your primary healthcare provider.

Neither the author nor the publisher shall be liable or responsible for any loss or damage allegedly arising from any information or suggestion in this book. Further, while every effort has been made to provide accurate contact information and Internet addresses at the time of publication, neither the author nor the publisher assumes any responsibility for errors, or for changes that occur after publication.

Edited by Roberta Tennant, MA. Editor-in-Chief at *Falcon Books*.
Designed by *Strategic Secrets* (www.strategicsecrets.com).

ISBN: 978-0-9973379-6-9 (Print)
ISBN: 978-0-9973379-9-0 (eBook)

Manufactured in the United States of America

This book is dedicated to my wonderful and supporting husband, Nelson Dockery. May the good Lord continue to give you a life of health, peace, and happiness.

Contents

Introduction
A Doctor on the Move to Positively Change Healthcare Outcomes

It has been more than twenty-five years of love, dedication, long hours at the office, stressful hospital rounds, some intimate home visits, but yet I felt the love and passion which I once had for medicine was slowly disappearing. As I began to reassess my purpose in life and ponder on my effectiveness as a physician to make lasting changes in the lives of my patients, I also began to ask myself the questions, why are so many people dying from diseases such as diabetes, hypertension, heart disease and cancer? How do we stop the epidemic of obesity and diabetes in our children. Surely if this trend continues our children's lifespan will be shorter than that of the parents. It is very obvious that we are living in an era of advanced medical science and in the United States of America we have the best hospitals, well-trained healthcare providers, and the most advanced technology, yet patients are sicker than they have ever been and thousands are dying daily from diseases that are not only preventable but also curable.

All these questions, conflicts and concerns propelled me on a different path to change the world around me. For me, it was no longer okay to prescribe pills to a young twenty-five-year-old patient who walked into my office with a blood pressure of

150/90, blood sugar of 250, and was overweight. This manner of practicing medicine was no longer the acceptable standard of care in my opinion. The prescription of medications alone without treating the root causes of the illnesses will not save lives. This is only a prescription for failure. During my over twenty-five years of practicing internal medicine I have seen too many lives destroyed as a result of diseases which are easily preventable with the integration of simple lifestyle changes.

Therefore, for the past several years I have integrated the GET HEALTHY FOR LIFE solution to empower my patients to change their health destiny. In this program, the emphasis is placed on educating, inspiring and empowering the patients to change lifestyle habits. This program addresses the root causes of diseases. Patients are instructed on how to make simple but effective changes that will not only lead to prevention but in many cases to patients experiencing disease reversal.

I can now truly say that my love for medicine has never been stronger. Now I spend much time working intimately with my patients, educating them on how to live their lives differently in order to prevent or reverse chronic diseases. The patients are now enjoying better health, they are happier and they now have a new lease on life. Just recently this seventeen-year-old young lady walked into my medical office for a routine visit. She was filled with excitement and happiness as she shouted, "Dr. Cooper, I lost five more pounds! I am now down twenty pounds since my initial visit, and now I will be beautiful for my prom." She continued to explain that her goal was to wear a beautiful dress that night. She then said to me,

"Hey, Dr. Cooper, I don't plan to become a lawyer anymore." I immediately inquired as to why the change? This is a young lady who would make a brilliant lawyer. She has the personality, she is intelligent and most importantly she loves to talk. I continued my conversation with her and asked why the change of heart? She said, "I have decided to be a nutritionist. I want to do what you are doing. I want to help people cure their disease." I became very emotional. My eyes were filled with tears, she was crying, and her sister and her mother who were present in the room were also crying. You see, this patient's story is much more profound. When she first came to me for treatment, she presented with her mother and sister. All three patients were overweight, and they had uncontrolled diabetes. This young lady said to me then, "Dr. Cooper, I am fat and I am not beautiful, but it is my goal to be beautiful for my high school prom." Her initial HbA1C was 9.5 (this is a test used to indicate how controlled a patient's blood sugar is. Normal is 4.0-6.0). Within a few weeks of implementing my GET HEALTHY FOR LIFE program, her blood sugar was controlled. The HbA1C was down to the normal range. The fact she was able to experience such significant change in her life influenced her desire to share in order to change the world. For me this is powerful! This is exactly the experience that I want you to have.

I am well aware that change is never easy. In fact, anything that is worth having will indeed require some sacrifice. As you continue to read this book you will be educated on various important subjects such as the impact that food, exercise, rest, healthy relationships and faith has on health and longevity. You will be empowered to change your health destiny as well as the lives of others. Some of the changes that you will need to make might be hard but not at all impossible. I know that making change is never easy, but it is important to note that determination, endurance, drive and perseverance will be needed to take you over the finish line.

Many of my patients have walked this path before you. Some have achieved more than others but they all are enjoying better health and happiness. Some of these patients have reduced their medications, and some have reversed diabetes, hypertension, and high cholesterol. Others have decreased pain and lost weight. They all for sure are enjoying much better health. As for me, I am delighted. I am excited because I am experiencing so many health miracles in the lives of my patients. I am a doctor on the move with the goal to positively change healthcare outcomes using lifestyle modifications, for all the people I am able to reach. Why don't you join the movement! My goal is to educate, inspire and empower you too!

G=Goal: Assess Your Health Risk and Establish Goals

Each passing year that we live our lives brings us new opportunities to better ourselves in some way. The excitement of a brand new year brings us hope to dream big, desire more out of our lives and envision new goals to help us achieve a brighter future. A common tradition at the beginning of every January is the New Year's resolution. Approximately one out of every three Americans takes part in this tradition and determines to better themselves in some way in the coming year. Unfortunately, a much smaller percentage of people actually follow through with their goals. A study conducted in 2002 found that 75% of people who set New Year's resolutions stick to the goals, but six months later, less than half are still on target at about 46%.[1]

New Year's resolutions and goal setting are commonplace in our society. So then why do we have such a high rate of failure so shortly after launch? Could it be that most people fail to take a comprehensive look at their situation(s) and carefully assess where they are in life and what they really want to achieve? In order to succeed at any goal, there must be a readiness to change.

The Cold Reality

According to polls, 66% of all the New Year's resolutions made in the country are associated with weight loss and improving one's health. This is followed by finances and financial status, then family and friends.[2] People are wanting to lose weight and live healthier lives. There's no surprise there. We all know that there are several benefits to losing weight:

- You feel better
- You look better
- Your overall health improves
- You have greater resistance to illnesses
- You have more energy and
- Your mood and attitude improve

With all these benefits, why is it that we have such a high fail rate when it comes to our own health? Two of the most common reasons why people abandon their New Year's resolutions are that they claim not to have enough time or "*it's too difficult.*" Those are the two most frequently used excuses as to why people abandon their goals to live and eat healthier. What is even more interesting (or alarming as it were) is the fact that 9 times out of 10, those same people had made the same resolutions some time before. Somehow, they let their dreams and their goals slip away from them. They lost sight of what they wanted out of life and ended up in a circle of complacency. As I counsel with others, whether they are my patients or just someone attending one of my seminars, I always mention that in order for them to succeed with their goals then a few things must happen. They must first assess their situation, then believe that there is a solution. The next step is taking action for change. Make this change a habit and live. You must believe, change and then live.

Everything is impossible - until it's done.

Prior to the 1940s people worldwide died from simple infections such as pneumonia, infection of the bladder and others. Doctors then had no effective forms of treatments. However, after many years of research and studies, Alexander Fleming discovered the magic cure, Penicillin. What was once seen as impossible is now simply a dream of the past. The discovery of Penicillin in the 1940s is seen as one of the greatest discoveries in the medical sciences. During his life, Leonardo da Vinci was considered a great artist and painter, but the 1800s was when the thousands of pages of writings and drawings that we collectively refer to today as Leonardo's codices began to surface. With the rediscovery of these documents, da Vinci was recast as a Renaissance visionary who saw the possible in the

7

world at a time when they were still considered "impossible" – things such as flight. Although it was envisioned in the 1800s, flight was still never achieved until December 17, 1903, in Kitty Hawk, North Carolina, when two brothers – Orville and Wilbur Wright – made the "impossible" a reality. They became the first people to ever develop a machine that was able to achieve controlled, sustained flight with a pilot aboard. Today, we see planes flying overhead and we think nothing of it. However, only a hundred years ago, this feat was considered "impossible".

There were many who tried to dampen the Wright brothers' determination to achieve their goal with mocking tones and discouraging words. Relentlessly, they persisted until finally, they made a breakthrough. Because of their resolve and tenacity to make their dreams and their goals a reality, they were able to do what everyone else was telling them couldn't be done. As a woman of faith, I ask that you permit me to leave this quote from the Bible. Matthew 19:26 says: "But Jesus beheld them, and said unto them, with men this is impossible, but with God all things are possible."

Dream Big

"Only big dreams have the power to move men's souls." This quote is from Marcus Aurelius – emperor of the great Roman Empire. He knew a fundamental truth about goals. That is, when you set your goals, you have to make them worth your while. If your goals do not move you, if they aren't enough to wake you up in the mornings, fill your mind through the day and infiltrate your dreams as you sleep, then what makes you think that you'll even remember them tomorrow? They have to be worth it and get you excited about it so that you can shake off those shackles of complacency and move into a position where you can create change. This is why goals fail – this is why dreams die. When a person sets a goal, it usually always involves additional work, risk or effort. In the business world there is a common understanding that there are minimal gains if the investor takes the minimum risk; however, the gains increase exponentially the higher the risk. If the dream is not worth it, then the goal will never happen – because it wasn't big enough. People set themselves up for failure by thinking too small. You have to dream big and then you'll spark a catalyst that can't be put out.

Anything in life worth having comes at a price. You need to be able to persist through the hardships in order to get where you want to be. By setting goals you are able to create in your mind an enduring vision. Every step you take along your journey – every obstacle that you overcome will invigorate you with short-term motivation which will turn into long-term success. Goals help to keep you focused and help you to organize your time and your resources so that you can make the most of your life.

A White-Hot Desire

Take a look at some of today's top-level athletes, successful doctors, lawyers, business people and achievers in all fields and walks of life. One thing that they all have in common is that they all set goals. But we are not just talking about small, short-term goals. Let's look at a top USA tennis champion, Serena Williams. She is a woman of determination; she works hard practice many hours daily. She is usually on the tennis court very early in the morning practicing for many hours of the day with one single focus and that is to win the next game. If you watch her on the field you will agree with me that she goes out with that same determination to fight to the end. Some games she wins but in other she struggles. However, to succeed at your goal, preparation, determination, fight, struggles, working hard and getting to the finish line are all part of achieving success. Sometimes with all the struggles, sacrifices, and tough choices that a person needs to endure in order to keep moving towards a goal, you might ask what keeps the motivation alive. The answer is a desire to succeed. Not just any type of desire but **white-hot** desire.

In the 1930s, Napoleon Hill coined the term white-hot desire and the reason that he used this analogy of 'white-hot' was that in the manufacturing plants which were common in those days, the temperature had to be so extreme that it glowed white.[3] The Bible refers to it as the refiner's fire that burns away the impurities. This is the power of the heat that is strong enough to purify and liquefy one of the earth's strongest elements. Now think about this concept for just a moment. That is the kind of burning desire that it takes to achieve your goals. This fire must be able to withstand the trials that you may have to face. It can't be just a little flame that can be put out with a strong wind. This fire must drive you with a white-hot desire that you feel in your core. It must fill you to the point where quitting is never an option.

How Setting Goals Affects Our Health

Now, there are things in everybody's life that give us a certain level of enjoyment. One of those things that most people can deeply and collectively appreciate is food. People celebrate important events and milestones by eating together.

Let's be honest, food gives pleasure. Every human wants to enjoy delicious food. However, it is absolutely vital to remember that what we put into our bodies is what fuels us. Believe it or not, most people take better care of their cars than their bodies. Let's be honest, would you put cooking oil in the gas tank? However, too many people use sugar or foods high in sodium and cholesterol to fuel their bodies. This eventually can lead to obesity, diabetes, heart disease and many other serious diseases. Many researchers are now confirming that the number one cause of chronic diseases and early death is related to poor food choices. Improving your health through the consumption of healthy food intake is a simple yet effective method of living with the quality of life that our Creator intended for us. Scientists and healthcare providers are now supporting plant-based foods as a better alternative to animal-based foods such as dairy, meats or cheese which are naturally higher in cholesterol.[4] A diet high in fruits, vegetables, nuts, seeds and whole grains will decrease the surge of obesity and other chronic diseases. Some people consider obesity as a cosmetic problem, but in fact, recent medical science and study are proving that it is more of a health problem. Obesity is indeed a disease, which leads to several life-threatening conditions and complications.

Some of the health consequences of poor nutrition are:

- Coronary Heart Disease
- Sleep apnea
- High blood pressure
- Metabolic syndrome
- Stroke
- Obesity

- Hypoventilation syndrome
- Osteoarthritis
- Reproductive problems
- Gallstones
- Type 2 Diabetes
- Cancer

Diabetes is one of the most widespread chronic diseases in the world today. It is an illness that affects the body's ability to use and break down sugars or glucose. Glucose is important because it is the main source of energy for our brain.[5] There are two main types of diabetes: type 1 and type 2. Also, there is a condition called pre-diabetes and it refers to a condition where the sugar level in your blood is higher than usual, but not high enough to be classified as diabetes. Some of the signs of diabetes are: increased thirst and increased need for food, frequent urination, and unexplained weight loss, the presence of ketones in your urine, fatigue, irritability, blurred vision, infections, and slow-healing sores.

One of the risk factors for diabetes is obesity. About 90% of people who are diagnosed with Type 2 diabetes are overweight.[6] Obesity can actually prevent our bodies from effectively using insulin in the transport of glucose from the blood to the cells, and thus maintain normal blood glucose levels. This phenomenon is referred to as insulin resistance. Diabetes is not a disease anyone wants to have. It can be a devastating disease. Today, over 9% of the population of the United States has diagnosed diabetes, and 25-27% has pre-diabetes. What is even more troubling is the fact that, according to the American Diabetes Association and Centers for Disease Control and Prevention, 1 in 4 of those people doesn't know.[7] That is 86 million people who are unaware that they have this chronic illness. Diabetes is a killer and is responsible for contributing to the deaths of over 234,051 people each year.[8] If you have diabetes then make it your goal to get rid of it!

Fortunately, there is hope. Diabetes can be prevented and even reversed with healthy lifestyle choices, like maintaining a healthy weight and having a proper diet consisting of plant-based foods. As little as 30 minutes of physical activity in your day can also greatly reduce your risk for diabetes and even possibly reverse it. Obesity is also associated with depression, anxiety and reduced energy levels. In addition to the physical ailments of obesity, there are several psychological effects as well. Self-confidence and self-esteem tend to plummet and anxiety levels rise as your weight rises. Only 10 pounds less can make a significant difference. Setting simple goals to control weight gain and taking steps to help reduce, prevent or reverse diabetes can make a world of difference for your health.

The Formula

Although goal setting is important, the reason for wanting to achieve goals as well as the methodology that is used to set those goals is equally as important. Just recently a young lady came to my office to establish care. She is a senior in high school, obviously very intelligent with the desire to become a lawyer. Unfortunately, she had diabetes and was obese, but she came in with very clear goals, to control her diabetes and to lose weight before her high school prom. She added that she wanted to be able to wear a very beautiful dress. We both agreed on the formula needed to achieve these goals, and she agreed to work hard.

I am delighted to report that this young lady has already controlled her diabetes, she has lost weight and she looks beautiful. She had specific goals, and she had a timeline outlined which led to early success. If your goals are vague or obscure – or likewise, if they are outrageous or foolish – then you will probably not find very much success along your journey and instead of becoming motivated to live and be better, you will end up discouraged, frustrated and all too often, unsatisfied with where you end up. *"I want to lose weight"* is a vague goal. You need to ask yourself defining questions such as:

- **How much weight do you want to lose?**
- **What is the time frame that you are giving yourself?**
- **How many pounds is that per month?**
- **How are you going to get there?**

These are all questions that you need to ask when you make the decision to set a goal. Improper goal setting can do more damage than it does good. But that is not to discourage you from wanting to achieve more. Think about setting sharp, clearly defined goals you can measure and take pride in the achievement of those goals, and you'll see forward progress in what might previously have seemed a long pointless grind. As you progress, you will also find your self-confidence rising as you recognize your own ability and competence in achieving the goals that you've set. Make sure that you write everything down. Writing your goals down makes them more tangible. It helps when you can see them every day. Put them on your fridge or in your office. Make sure that you have daily reminders about what it is you are working for.

Setting and achieving goals does not happen overnight. It can sometimes take many days, weeks, even months to find or plan a path that will help us to be the person that we want to see in the mirror. Goal setting is a process.

You can set your goals on a number of levels:

- *First, you create your "big picture" of what you want to do with your life (or over, say, the next 10*

15

years), and identify the large-scale goals that you want to achieve.

- *Then, you break these down into the smaller and smaller targets that you must hit to reach your lifetime goals.*
- *Once you have your plan, you start working on it to achieve these goals.*
- *Celebrate and Reward yourself as you succeed with the goals you have established.*

As you start working towards the things that you want to achieve in your life, you will find confidence in yourself with every obstacle that you overcome. You will start to feel better about yourself and others will notice the difference in you. Your attitude will start to change as you find more and more motivation to become successful. Work down to the things that you can do in, say, the next five years, then next year, next month, next week, and today, to start moving towards them with a focused ambition.

"... A Single Step"

Short-term goals are usually the easiest place to start when creating a plan of action. Goal setting is a powerful process for thinking about what you want your future to look like and where you want to be further along down the road, but even though you may have big dreams, it is always a good idea to start small and grow from there. A tree does not become a tree overnight. It starts off as a seed. With water, sunlight and an enriching environment, it starts to push its way through the soil, or cement, or anything that stands in its way. Soon it starts to sprout its branches towards Heaven and becomes a tree. Short-term goals are a good way to help keep us focused and motivated to continue on. They also help by keeping the big picture at the back of your mind as daily reminders of what you are working towards. By knowing precisely what you want to achieve, you know where you have to concentrate your efforts.

'Pressing Matters'

In today's society, it often feels as though we are being pulled in every direction. Life gets so busy with so many 'pressing matters' that we tend to forget what really *matters*. You see, 'pressing matters' don't always *matter*. You have to make sure that you make time for those things that really *matter*. Things like faith, family, friends, our health – the gifts of God. That is what people tend to forget. Driven by financial and professional success people oftentimes lose focus on the little things that are the most important to us. When setting goals – whatever they may be – do not neglect the things that matter.

Help along the way

I can do all things through Him who strengthens me.
-Philippians 4:13

17

For some people, their goal is to lose weight, for others, it might be to get into a better financial position and for others, it could be to grow in their faith. Whatever the final desired outcome is, setting goals will make the process smoother. Sometimes, however, you might feel as if you're getting nowhere – as if you've hit an immovable obstacle in the road. Sometimes you may feel that for all your struggles and all your tears and all your heartache, you are not making one bit of difference. That is the time when we must come to the throne and remember: "For we wrestle not against flesh and blood, but against principalities, against powers, against the rulers of the darkness of this world, against spiritual wickedness in high places." - Ephesians 6:12

When we become disheartened and we feel that we cannot go on by ourselves, this can create feelings of depression, frustration, and anger. These feelings are completely contrary to what the Bible says that God wants us to be. We know that there is someone who is willing to carry us through. Remember that the fruits of the Spirit are love, joy, peace, patience, kindness, goodness, faithfulness, gentleness and self-control. - Galatians 5:22-23.

In Summary

Goal setting is a powerful process for thinking about what your expectations for the future would be and how you plan to achieve success. If the Wright brothers never had a goal in mind that they were pursuing, do you think that they would have ever accomplished what they did? Humans had dreamt of flight since da Vinci. What do you think was the difference? Da Vinci was a great Renaissance man — with his incredible paintings and his marvelous mind. However, the Wright brothers are known for only one thing. They had their eyes, their hearts, focused on one goal — flight. They made a place for themselves in history because of their steadfast determination in achieving their goal.

Goals will drive you to turn your vision into a reality. If you are reading this book then maybe your goal is to achieve freedom from disease whether physical or mental, or it may be that you want to learn how to protect yourself or family from the cold hands of chronic illnesses or death. However, whatever the case, careful planning, taking appropriate steps, and making sacrifices are the keys to your success.

2

E- Environment: Spend Time in the Outdoors. Enjoy Natural Healing From the Sunlight and Fresh Air

According to scientists, the distance from Earth to the Sun is 92,955,807 miles which is measured in what is called an astronomical unit, or AU. The AU is used to measure distances throughout the solar system. We have found through technology and science that this distance creates the perfect balance of cooling and heating to support life here on Earth – making it thrive as the planet we can all enjoy today. Let's look at the various gasses that make up the atmosphere, nitrogen 78%, oxygen 20%, carbon dioxide .04%. This makeup is just right to sustain life. Water is another important element that is abundant in our environment. It is essential to maintain good health and to sustain life.

Did you know that the sunshine also gives life? All these elements, water, air, and sunlight, give healing and longevity. Life, as we currently know it, can flourish only in a suitable environment. It requires an appropriate balance of climate, water, land, and air. As members of this planet, it is important to understand that *our* health, as human beings, is also affected by any changes in our environment as well as the rest of the flora and fauna that co-exists along with us. Changes in our environment, such as pollution and destruction of natural wildlife and vegetation, can have a negative impact on human life.

A healthy environment is one of the most important aspects of our survival, yet far too many of us take it for granted – even the very air that we breathe. Forests cover 31 percent of the world's land surface. That is an estimated 4 billion hectares. One hectare is equivalent to 2.47 acres. During the pre-industrial area, 5.9 billion hectares of forest covered the earth.[2] I'm sure that we are all aware that trees absorb carbon dioxide, which is poisonous to humans, and produce oxygen which we need to breathe and ultimately live. This balance allows us to live in harmony with our environment where each one's existence benefits the other. We exhale carbon dioxide for the plants and they produce oxygen for us. It's a win-win situation.

Obtaining adequate amounts of fresh air gives life. A person cannot live without oxygen for more than 5 minutes; however, contaminated air can slowly rob you of good health. So then why are we destroying our forests? Not only that, but we are also polluting the very air that we all breathe. I recently saw on the news where the air pollution in China was so bad people were using face masks for protection. The exposure to toxic substances in the air leads to fatigue, lung disease, poor health, and cancer. Air pollution has become one of the biggest environmental concerns in recent years. Numerous governmental agencies are working to try to decrease and possibly even reverse the damage that has been done and is currently being done to the Ozone layer. However, our lifestyles continue to destroy it at a rapid rate, let's look at tobacco smoking. For years that has been a great public health issue. Smoking is linked to the production of cancer of the lungs, the mouth, and throat, cancer of the bladder as well as diseases such as emphysema, heart disease, and poor circulation. For many years this poor lifestyle habit has led to so many health issues. It is great to finally know that statistics now show that the incidence of smoking is trending down.

The Greater Light to Rule the Day

According to the Christian Bible, "And God saw everything that He had made, and, behold, it was good." The "good" that is mentioned here is not just the regular "good" as we would normally presume. It goes much deeper than that to cover an all-encompassing and intrinsic meaning of the word. "Good" here in this sense is derived from the Hebrew word towb (tobe). According to Strong's Concordance Hebrew Lexicon, "good" or towb can be described as an adjective in the widest sense, used likewise as a noun, both in the masculine and the feminine, the singular and the plural.[4]

23

The functionality of the relationships of life here on this planet is so intertwined that without the health of one, another will suffer. For example, sunlight causes the brain to release the hormone serotonin which enhances mood. Exposure to sunlight helps to reduce depression and anxiety and can even lower our blood pressure and help to prevent hypertension. A team of British researchers found out that the nitric oxide which is stored in the upper layers of our skin reacts to sunlight and makes the blood vessels wider to allow the oxide to enter our bloodstream while also infusing us with the beneficial Vitamin D.[5] Vitamin D helps our bodies fight against illnesses such as tuberculosis, develop healthy bones and prevent osteoporosis and other bone diseases.[6] Vitamin D is also a pro-hormone which functions as a gene modulator, thus preventing the formation of cancer producing genes. Adequate amounts of vitamin D is also important for insulin to function effectively and thus reduce the risk of developing diabetes. It is very obvious then that adequate exposure to sunlight is important for health and longevity. Getting 10-15 minutes of exposure to the sun daily will produce your daily recommended dose of vitamin D, which is 1,000-2,000 IU.

The Harmful Effects of Air Pollution on Our Minds and Bodies

Air pollution is by far one of the most harmful forms of pollution in our environment due to the fact that it affects every living thing on such a rudimentary basis. Air pollution is one of the largest contributors to many cardiovascular and respiratory health issues that are evident today. Some of the main causes of air pollution are the pollutants emitted by motor vehicles and power plants and factories. Gasses like sulfur dioxide and nitrogen dioxide increase the symptoms of heart and lung conditions by irritating the airways. The particles that are released into the air from sources such as vehicle exhaust and other pollutants go deep into the lungs and can cause inflammation. Carbon monoxide prevents the intake of oxygen into the blood stream, decreasing the blood-oxygen levels. Evidence of increasing air pollution is seen in illnesses such as lung cancer, asthma, allergies, and various breathing problems along with severe and irreparable damage to flora and fauna. Even the most natural phenomenon of migratory birds has been hindered, with severe air pollution preventing them from reaching their seasonal metropolitan destinations.

In addition to respiratory and cardiovascular health risks, air pollution also has a negative impact on our mental and emotional health as well. Research conducted by the assistant professor of internal medicine at Rush Medical College, Jennifer Weuve, MPH, ScD, has shown that women between the ages of 70 and 81 who lived in an environment with polluted air suffered from a greater cognitive decline than the women at the same age who live in a less polluted environment. Approximately 19,000 women were examined during this study.

The impact of air pollution is even taking its toll on our children and young adults. Shakira Franco Suglia, ScD, an assistant professor at Boston University's School of Public Health, found that children who are exposed to these higher levels of air pollution scored lower on tests of memory and verbal and nonverbal IQ than those who were not. Cognitive skills are not the only symptoms of air pollution. Children who are exposed to higher levels of urban air pollutants such as polycyclic aromatic hydrocarbons suffer from additional symptoms of depression and anxiety. This evidence was further proved by the research done by Frederica Perera, DrPH, at the Columbia University Mailman School of Public Health where children from New York, ages ranging from about 6 to 7 years old, were the subjects.

Tobacco and the Hazards of Second-Hand Smoke

An experiment was conducted in north Italy to determine what kind of an impact various pollutant sources had on the particulate levels of the air. The test was conducted with a diesel engine as one subject and filtered cigarettes as the other. A turbo diesel two-liter engine fueled with low sulfur fuel, was started and left idling for 30 minutes in a test garage with the garage door closed. Afterward, the doors were left open for 4 hours. Three filtered cigarettes were then lit up in sequence and left lit for an additional 30 minutes. The nicotine and tar content of each cigarette was 1 mg and 11.2 mg, respectively. A portable analyzer took readings every two minutes during the experiments. Combined particulate levels in the first hour after the engine had been started measured 88 ug / m3.

Those recorded in the first hour after the cigarettes had been lit measured 830 ug / m3. The result was that the particulate level of the subject area was 10 times greater with the cigarettes than just the diesel engine alone. Although the diesel engine exhaust doubled the particulate matter levels found outdoors at its peak, the environmental tobacco smoke particulate matter reached levels 15 times greater than those measured outdoors.[7]

The Painted World

Colors also have an impact on our health. The colors that we experience today are no accident. It is a known fact that light levels and colors have a significant effect on people. During the day, it has been found that even indoor lighting conditions that mimic daylight stimulate hormone production which increases a persons' alertness and activity throughout the day – specifically, blue light, at about 460 nm. Cognitive performance is better and concentration is improved. Warmer color temperatures later on in the evenings are preferred to assist in the production of melatonin which is the hormone secreted from the pineal gland that is needed for sleep. By getting better sleep and promoting a balanced circadian rhythm, people reduce their stress and anxiety levels, which stimulates positive health, behavior, and overall productivity. Although this is not commonly practiced some researchers recommend certain lighting levels for senior citizens because scientists are finding that color has more of an impact than we previously anticipated. Studies have shown that subjects whose average age was 85 demonstrated improvements in depression, agitation, and sleep when they received high daytime levels of light.[8]

Good Like Medicine

Technology and science today have allowed us to measure the dangers of pollution on our physical and even mental health. We, as logical beings, can't argue this fact because we have the numbers, studies and statistics reinforced by evidence-based research to prove the point. However, there are other environmental factors that can affect the health of an individual which are just as obvious, but not always as recognized. Our environment at home and the people we surround ourselves with can also affect our health. It is believed that about 40 percent of people who are diagnosed with depression can trace it back to a genetic link. Environmental and other factors make up the other 60 percent.[9]

What are these environmental factors? Our family and friends, whom we choose to associate with and allow around us and our loved ones. There is a saying: "Misery loves company." This is actually very true. Chris Segrin, a professor of Psychology and Communications at the University of Arizona in Tucson, found that people who were exposed to severely depressed subjects over an extended period of time experienced a decline in mood over a six-week period. When the subjects spent time away, they noticeably cheered up. Although this study was specifically targeting depressive moods, Segrin's results were the same for people with sunny dispositions. The positive and happy subjects increased the moods of those who surrounded them.[10] In addition, laughter is good for the soul and it has been proven that even our physiology changes when we laugh. Our pulse and blood pressure go up, and we breathe faster, sending more oxygen to our tissues. As a matter of fact, the effects of laughter and exercise are very similar. William Fry, a laughter research pioneer, claimed that it took him a ten-minute workout on a rowing machine for his heart rate to reach the same level that it did after just one minute of genuine laughter. Other benefits of laughter include immune response, relaxation, and sleep – even blood sugar levels.

In fact, 19 people with diabetes were a part of a study that looked at the effects of laughter on blood sugar levels. The group was directed to attend a tedious lecture after first eating a meal. The very next day, the same group of 19 people ate the exact same meal and then watched a comedy. The group's blood sugar levels were recorded before and after both the lecture and the comedy on both days and what the researchers found was very impressive. The groups' blood sugar levels were lower after the comedy, than they were after the lecture.[11] There is an ancient proverb that says, "A merry heart doeth good like a medicine: but a broken spirit drieth the bones."

The Importance of Our Social Structures

The support of others is also a very important aspect of health. In fact, one study revealed that women suffering from breast cancer who took part in support group sessions once every week survived twice as long as those ladies who did not. According to Erik Peper, Ph.D., Associate Director of the Institute for Holistic Healing Studies at San Francisco State University, "There is overwhelming evidence that people who have few social contacts are more likely to get sick and less likely to recover from an illness."

Social relationships can also have an impact on people who suffer from clinical depression. A research study done by the University of Michigan in 2013 showed that one of the risk factors for becoming depressed is the *quality* of the relationships people have with one another. Moreover, some unconventional treatments for some cases of clinical depression that have had considerable results have been to spend time with positive people, take care of animals, and to help others in need.

According to Dr. Richard Schulze, helping others has been known to benefit people who suffer from heart disease, neurological conditions, emotional disorders such as depression, anxiety, stress-related conditions and even cancer.

Humans are social creatures. Our first social structures are our families and from there, we branch out to friends, acquaintances, co-workers and so forth. These important social structures help us to build strong mental and psychological bonds with both our inner selves and our world. They teach us things such as articulate speech, which is a gift reserved for mankind alone. No other creature on earth can boast this gift except human beings. One of the most crippling conditions of feral children who were raised without such structures or social support is the inability to communicate articulately. We also learn appropriateness and how to cope and deal with difficult realities such as death or loss through these social channels. It was never intended for a person to have to walk through life alone. When God created Adam He followed up with Eve right after and placed them in the Garden of Eden, a perfect environment which would have supported a life without diseases or death had it not been for the fall of man. He said that it was not good that man be alone. Our environment matters – and it's not just how it affects us on the outside, but also how it affects us on the inside.

3

T = Timely Rest: Restore, Repair, and Rejuvenate During Sleep

On June nineteenth, 2015, a truck driver by the name of Mark Tipton, age 52, failed to stop in a construction zone and caused a chain-reaction crash involving his Freightliner and 12 other vehicles at 3:50 a.m. on the inbound lanes of Interstate 55 in Illinois. All inbound lanes of the expressway were closed for about two hours and Mark admitted to police that he did not even attempt to stop or slow down. He was going full speed in his semi-truck because he had fallen asleep at the wheel. Sleep deprivation is one of the main causes of vehicular accidents in the United States. In fact, The National Highway Transportation Safety Administration (NHTSA) estimates that as many as 100,000 accidents are caused by drivers who actually doze off behind the wheel of their vehicles. It is also estimated that as many as 1,500 deaths and 40,000 injuries may be caused by drowsy driving.[1] According to a recent study conducted by the Sleep Medicine division at Harvard Medical School, over fifty percent of participants admitted to driving while drowsy. Another twenty-five percent revealed they had actually fallen asleep at the wheel even if it was only momentarily. The statistics for semi-truck drivers were even more alarming with nearly half of them admitting to actually 'drifting off' while driving over-the-road.[2] The lack of adequate sleep will surely take your life or the life of others, whether during a motor vehicle accident or not. Adequate sleep is essential for good health. An inadequate amount of restful sleep not only leads to poor health but to death. It is, for this reason, timely rest is listed as one of the pillars of health. It is a well-known fact that oxygen and water are essential to sustain life, but have you ever to stopped to think where sleep falls in that formula for life sustenance? Let's look in more detail: How long could you sustain life in the absence of the following:

1. Oxygen – five minutes.
2. Sleep – three to possibly eleven days
3. Water – seven to ten days
4. Food – fourteen to twenty-one days.

Timely Rest Is Made Law

On July 1st, 2013, the U.S. Department of Transportation's Federal Motor Carrier Safety Administration (FMCSA) announced that new federal regulations designed to improve safety for the motoring public by reducing truck driver fatigue would take full effect. This legislation passed due to the increase in motor vehicle accidents as a result of drowsy driving. Drowsy driving is very similar to driving while under the influence of drugs or alcohol. In fact, one study found that driving after being awake for seventeen to eighteen hours is equivalent to driving with a blood alcohol content of 0.05 percent.[4] People who are sleep deprived experience symptoms such as:

- Impaired coordination
- Slow reaction times
- Impaired judgment
- Decreased vision

The FMCSA estimates that the new safety regulations will save nineteen lives and prevent approximately 1,400 crashes and 560 injuries each year.[3] The importance of proper and adequate rest is not only essential for drivers, but for everyone. The human body and mind require a certain amount of rest so that they are able to perform the everyday activities and processes that we need them to. If we do not get enough sleep, we will be less productive and our moods will change, normally for the worse. Healthy sleep is essential for providing energy enough for the next day and also for processing and retaining information.

Can A Lack of Sleep Affect Our Memory?

There is no question that sleep, or a lack thereof, affects a person's brain, but to what extent? Is there a greater chance to memorize the things we learn before we go to sleep? According to recent studies, the answer is "yes." Sleep can actually trigger changes in the brain that solidify memory by strengthening the connections between brain cells and transferring information from one brain region to another. Researchers did a test on a group of subjects who had learned new material or skills, such as practicing piano scales, and then scanned their brains after a period both with and without sleep. They found that the regions of the brain that control speed and accuracy were more active in those people who had slept than those who hadn't. People who have a good night's sleep or even just take a nap after they learn something are more likely to retain that information on a long-term basis.[5] Scientists believe that while we sleep, memories and skills are shifted to more efficient and permanent brain regions, making for higher proficiency the next day. Sleep is also known to increase creative ability.

Further research has found that there is a possibility that the human brain can learn during periods of sleep as well. In an experiment, scientists exposed a group of people to a sound and a pleasant smell while they slept. After the subjects woke up in the morning, they started sniffing when they heard the sound. In other words, they had learned the association in their sleep.

Working in the U.S.A

Although it cannot buy happiness, money is an important means of achieving a higher quality of life. The United States ranks high on the charts as far as housing, income and wealth are concerned. The average household income per capita is $41,355 a year, which is the highest figure according to the Organization for Economic Cooperation and Development. We rank above the average in health status, jobs and earnings, personal security and environmental quality but below average in the work/life balance.[6] As Americans, our economy and consequently our nation is driven by business. The general cultural expectation in the U.S. remains the traditional "nine to five," but it is increasingly common for most employees to work beyond this point. While eight hours per day is often the "official" expectation, many employees feel they need to work longer.

In many industries and regions, over twelve hours per day has become the normal working timeframe. Even when not at work, employees tend to "be on call" with the increase in technology such as email, smartphones, and the Internet. Working long daily and weekly hours on a continuing basis seems normal to most of us; however, these types of lifestyle patterns are associated with a number of serious chronic health conditions such as chronic fatigue, a weakened immune system, mental disorders, anxiety and even auditory and visual hallucinations just to name a few.

The Importance of Rest and Relaxation

The United States is the only developed country in the world without a single, legally required paid vacation or holiday. By

37

law, every country in the European Union has at least four work weeks of paid vacation.[7] Because time-off is time not spent productively working, it would seem to be an expense that countries with struggling economies cannot afford. However, countries such as Germany and France offer about the highest amount of paid time off and were only marginally lower as far as macroeconomic outcomes were concerned than the U.S. Another important note that we must also consider is the fact that the average U.S. employee works approximately twenty percent more hours per worker than employees in Germany or France.

Fight-or-Flight

I think that it is fair to say that everyone can appreciate an honest day's work; however, overworking oneself can actually do more harm than good. Constant stages of work and stress can deteriorate the body at a rapid rate. In the 1930s, a scientist by the name of Hans Selye applied the term "stress" to living organisms and their struggle to live, cope and adapt to their changing environments. One of his most significant discoveries was that the stress hormone cortisol had a long-term effect on the health of rats.[8] Traditionally, cortisol has played a dynamic role in human survival. We have all heard of the infamous "fight-or-flight" reaction. This is when a hostile situation is deduced by our brains and a chain reaction of signals releases various hormones such as epinephrine, which is also known as "adrenaline," norepinephrine, and cortisol from the adrenal glands. These resources cause a physiological response to that threat in the form of increased heart rate and faster breathing, and increase the availability of glucose, which fuels our cells. These responses take so much energy that they leave few resources for the other important functions that are necessary for our health. As a result, the hormone cortisol will simultaneously tell other costly physical processes – including digestion, reproduction, physical growth, and some aspects of the immune system – to shut or slow down until the threat passes so that they do not interfere with the defense process from the imminent danger that is presumed.

Adrenal Fatigue

The hormones that cause "stress" are important aspects of survival; however, continuous release of them is hazardous to the body because the results are very taxing. Sometimes, when stress levels go on for extended periods of time, the brain can perceive stress even if it isn't really there. Adrenal fatigue is a decrease in the adrenal glands' ability to carry out their normal functions. It is commonly caused by chronic stress from any source including emotional, physical, mental, or environmental that exceeds the body's capacity to adjust appropriately to the demands for more and more cortisol. Stressors that can lead to adrenal fatigue include anger, chronic illness, depression, high sugar intake and sleep deprivation, just to name a few. Moreover, chronic stress and a prolonged exposure to cortisol inhibit the growth of new neurons in the hippocampus, a brain area essential in forming new memories. In this way, stress directly results in memory impairments and impairs the brain's ability to put emotional memories into context. It can cause increased growth of the amygdala, the portion of the brain that controls fear and other emotional responses.[9]

There are four main phases of adrenal fatigue. The first is the "alarm" phase where the body tries to compensate for the over-production of cortisol and posts a forceful anti-stress response to overcome it. In the second phase, the adrenal glands are eventually unable to keep up with the body's cortisol demand and although normal daily functions can still be carried out, the body will be exhausted after each day and will require more rest than usual in order to recover properly. If proper rest is not obtained, then the output of cortisol will gradually decline and the primary goal of the body will be to conserve energy. Energy sources such as muscle tissue are drained and used as fuel in order to ensure survival. At this point, people often cannot function smoothly throughout the day, no matter how hard they try.

In stage three of adrenal fatigue or the resistant phase, the endocrine system continues to focus on producing stress hormones at the expense of sex hormones. This then causes a drop in the level of hormones such as DHEA and testosterone. People who find themselves in this phase of adrenal fatigue will experience lower levels of many important hormones that can make a significant difference to the quality of life that they experience. Typical symptoms might include regular tiredness, a lack of enthusiasm, recurring infections and a lower sex drive. This phase might continue for several months or even years. The fourth and final stage of adrenal fatigue is the most dangerous and can sometimes be life-threatening. Addison's disease is a disorder that occurs when your body no longer produces sufficient doses of cortisol and oftentimes, it produces inadequate levels of aldosterone as well. Over time, a person can experience symptoms of Addisonian crisis when the body is completely exhausted. Such symptoms include chronic fatigue and muscle weakness, loss of appetite, the inability to digest food, weight loss, blood sugar abnormalities, including dangerously low blood sugar or hypoglycemia, low blood pressure, dizziness, fainting, nausea, vomiting, and diarrhea, moodiness, irritability, and depression.[10]

Can A Lack Of Sleep Make Me Gain Weight?

Traditionally, sleep has been regarded for its effects on the brain and emotions; however, research is showing us that even moderate sleep deprivation in healthy subjects can alter the person's metabolic state. This change is so significant because it literally mimics the glucose metabolism of diabetics. Going for extended periods of time without sufficient sleep can raise cortisol levels and decrease a person's insulin sensitivity. Another study showed that after four hours of sleep for six nights, healthy young men experienced a thirty percent decrease in their body's ability to metabolize carbohydrates. Scientists are starting to believe that there may be a connection between a lack of sleep and the obesity crisis that our country is currently facing.

Obesity affects over two-thirds, which is 68.8 percent, of adults in the United States. Although this statistic is incredibly alarming, what is even more alarming is the fact that this crisis is even affecting our future generations. About one-third of children and adolescents ages six to nineteen are considered to be overweight or obese. Four out of five people with type two diabetes, which contributes to the death of 234,051 Americans annually, are overweight or obese.[11]

What and How

Now that we have established the importance of sleep and what can happen to our bodies when we deprive ourselves of adequate rest, we are faced with the question of how much sleep is just right. To put it plainly, there is no secret formula or a one-size-fits-all approach. Every person is created differently and has different needs. However, scientists and researchers have come up with a very basic formula of approximately eight hours of sleep per night for optimal cognitive performance. Although the "eight-hour rule" is the general guideline, each person's age plays a significant role in how their sleeping patterns should be tailored. For example, anyone who has had children knows that eight hours of sleep each night is only a dream with infants. The National Sleep Foundation recommends that newborns typically get between fourteen to seventeen hours of sleep each day.[12] Because they usually require scheduled feedings, however, newborn babies will typically take naps in one to three hour intervals to get their essential levels of sleep time. After infancy, the amount of time necessary for each age bracket is reduced by about two hours until the eight hour mark is reached at adulthood and remains that way into the senior citizen status. Here is a further breakdown of the daily recommended hours of sleep according to the National Sleep Foundation:

- Newborns (0-3 months): Sleep range narrowed to 14-17 hours each day (previously it was 12-18)
- Infants (4-11 months): Sleep range widened two hours to 12-15 hours (previously it was 14-15)
- Toddlers (1-2 years): Sleep range widened by one hour to 11-14 hours (previously it was 12-14)
- Preschoolers (3-5): Sleep range widened by one hour to 10-13 hours (previously it was 11-13)
- School-age children (6-13): Sleep range widened by one hour to 9-11 hours (previously it was 10-11)
- Teenagers (14-17): Sleep range widened by one hour to 8-10 hours (previously it was 8.5-9.5)
- Younger adults (18-25): Sleep range is 7-9 hours (new age category)
- Adults (26-64): Sleep range did not change and remains 7-9 hours
- Older adults (65+): Sleep range is 7-8 hours (new age category)

As with each individual, every slumber is not the same. There are phases of sleep that people slip into that provide for the healing and building processes and mental clarity that we have discussed thus far. The term "deep sleep" is the type of sleep where the restoration and growth of body tissue occur and immunity to infections is strengthened. Electroencephalo-graphic recordings are recordings that monitor brain activity during a person's sleep in measured wavelengths. The phases of sleep are characterized by wave-like formations that scale up and down in depths. The more brain activity, the greater the formation depths. Rapid-eye-movement sleep is a "deep sleep" where the brain activity actually resembles conscious-ness or wakefulness. As the name implies, during this phase of the sleeping cycle, both eyes move under closed eyelids as if watching or following fast moving objects. This is where dreaming, sleepwalking, and teeth-grinding occur. Mem-ory organization and re-organization, as well as the refresh-ing of memories, also take place in this phase of sleep. Rap-id-eye-movement sleep is the last and deepest sleep phase.[13]

Getting a Better Sleep

There are a few things that we can do to ensure that we are getting the proper sleep and rest levels that our bodies need to function properly and have enough energy to help us success-fully complete each new day.

- We should try to adhere to a timely sleep schedule. Consistency has been proven to reinforce the body's sleep-wake cycle and help promote a better quality of sleep at night. Try to be in bed by 10:00 PM. The hours prior to midnight allow for more production of the growth hormones. This, therefore, increases the processes of healing and reparation.

- Have a bedtime ritual. Do something that will relax you before going to bed so that you can easily drift off. Forcing yourself to sleep tends to have the opposite effect as it can add stress. Also, warm colored light such as those with a yellowish glow has been known to influence feelings of rest and relaxation in the brain, helping it to unwind.

- Daytime naps can interfere with proper nighttime rest. If naps are absolutely necessary or you find yourself utterly exhausted, you should limit your naps to last only between ten and thirty minutes.

- Physical activity such as walking, jogging or even simple house-cleaning can help you sleep better at night. In addition to the other numerous health benefits, physical activity can help you fall into a deeper sleep by expending any unused energy that accumulates throughout the day. One thing to remember though is not to exercise too close to bedtime. Try to exercise in the morning or afternoon, because exercising right before going to bed may keep you too energized to fall asleep.[14]

- Many people consider stress as the number one reason for not having a quality sleep. There are several ways that you can help to manage stress. Physical activity helps to alleviate stress and the over-production of cortisol during the day which will contribute to better sleep at night. Another good practice is to keep work from interfering with your personal life. Keeping work and home-life separate can greatly increase your chances of falling soundly asleep. Remember, tomorrow is another day. Do not worry about things that you cannot change and always move forward.
- Prayer, meditation, and giving thanks for all the day's blessings will allow for a good night's sleep.

In Summary

Please remember that in order for you to attain health and longevity there are two cycles of rest that must be observed: daily and weekly rest. This allows the body to restore and repair damaged cells, tissues and organs. Even God rested at the end of creation week, on the seventh day. He blessed it and made it holy and asked us to do the same. With so much to do and often, not enough time to do it in, we forget about our health as we focus on what all needs to be done. We tend to overthink and overwork ourselves without even noticing the damage we are doing to our bodies and our minds. Although it sometimes proves very difficult, keeping our daily lives organized will help to ensure that we make time for the important things such as our rest, our family, friends, and most importantly, our faith. By following the simple principles and practices of regular rest time like the Bible says we should, we will be able to live longer and healthier lives. We will find more peace and tranquility through the hectic hustle and bustle of each day and we will learn to have serenity in our lives as we were created to. Remember, *it is important to take time to rest, repair, rejuvenate, recharge, and refocus. This is a successful strategy for health.*

4

H-Healthy Diet: Healing with the Right Foods

Scurvy is a now a rare disease and the incidences of this condition are rather low, but in the 1600s and 1700s, it was a major medical concern – especially for sailors who navigated long voyages. Throughout history, scurvy was a painful disease that inflicted sailors with devastating symptoms such as loose teeth, loss of appetite, diarrhea, fever, numbness, skin lesions, internal hemorrhaging and occasional paralysis. As a matter of fact, it was not uncommon for those afflicted with the disease to perish. While serving as surgeon on HMS Salisbury, a Scottish naval surgeon named James Lind carried out experiments to discover the cause of scurvy and potentially, a remedy. Finally, in 1747, he found one. Lind discovered that sailors afflicted with scurvy who were fed citrus fruits experienced a remarkable recovery from the disease.[1] In fact, scurvy could be prevented altogether by including citrus fruits in the sailors' diets.

Another disease that afflicted sailors was beriberi – a degenerative disease with symptoms such as weight loss, body weakness and pain, brain damage, irregular heart rate, heart failure, and death if left untreated. In the 1880s, beriberi reached epidemic proportions in the Dutch colonies. Christiaan Eijkman was a Dutch physician who was serving in the Dutch colonial army as an army surgeon in the Dutch East Indies in exchange for his education as a physician. Toward the end of the nineteenth century, Eijkman traced the cause of the disease to diets that included polished and processed white rice rather than unpolished brown rice.[2]

In 1906, the British biochemist Sir Frederick Gowland Hopkins demonstrated that food contained what he called "accessory factors," but it wasn't until the chemist Casimir Funk found the vital substance that Eijkman called the anti-beriberi factor that the true cure was identified. Funk gave it the name "Vitamine." He coined the word by combining "vital" and "amine." This name later came to denote all vitamins and was accepted by the scientific community in 1912. Casimir Funk is considered to be the "father of vitamin therapy" to this day.[3]

What Does It All Mean?

Vitamins are organic nutrients which are present in food in small quantities, but in the 1800s, no one had ever heard of vitamins. As a result, scurvy was caused by a lack of ascorbic acid or Vitamin C in a person's food intake and beriberi was caused by a lack of Thiamine or Vitamin B1 which was lost in the polished white rice but was plentiful in natural brown rice grains. Hopkins' discovery was a major shift in our understanding of the importance of nutrition and Funk showed us that vitamins are essential to maintain our health, yet on a global scale nearly two billion people are vitamin-deficient with at least half of children worldwide ages 6 months to 5 years suffering from one or more micronutrient deficiencies according to the CDC (Centers for Disease Control and Prevention).[4]

Vitamins and minerals are often referred to as micronutrients. You only need small quantities of them in order to stay healthy, yet, if a person should fail to get the required amounts, disease and illness are virtually guaranteed. Micronutrients provide for the body's development, function, disease prevention, and over-all well-being. Although there are a few micronutrients that the body can produce on its own, most of them are not produced in sufficient quantities to sustain us without dietary contributions. They **must** be derived from the food that we eat. In developed countries, it is estimated that the average adult eats approximately six hundred grams of food per day. Less than one gram of that food consists of vitamins.[5] Inadequate nutrient intake results in deficiency disorders and diseases such as beriberi and scurvy.

Nutrients

We have all heard the term nutrients or nutrition or some other variation of the word. Due to recent trends, people are becoming a lot more conscious of the kinds of foods that they are eating; however, people are still becoming ill and aging and dying prematurely. We are still seeing diseases such as diabetes and obesity climb to all-time highs at an alarming rate — faster than they ever have before. How can this be? There are a lot of myths that surround this topic and a lot of false information. In an effort to combat these issues, we are going to break down the subject into easy to digest sections... pun intended.

Nutrients are substances in foods that provide energy and materials for cell development, growth, and repair. There are six kinds of nutrients in food:[5]

- carbohydrates
- proteins
- fats & lipids
- vitamins
- minerals
- water

Carbohydrates, proteins, vitamins, and fats are all organic nutrients and can be broken down quite easily by heat, air, or acid. Unfortunately, due to their characteristics, cooking, storage, and even simple exposure to air can inactivate these fragile compounds. On the other hand, minerals and water are inorganic and have a more robust chemical structure and can withstand more exposure.[6] It is also interesting to note that, unlike carbohydrates, proteins, vitamins, and fats which are made up of two or more molecules, minerals are stand-alone compounds that appear on the Periodic Table of Elements. Nutritionists and other healthcare providers determine the recommended daily amount or RDA of a nutrient by how much each body needs it to stay healthy. Nutrients can be obtained in a variety of ways ranging from dietary choices to supplemental intake. A nutritional deficiency is when the body doesn't absorb the necessary amount of a particular nutrient.[7]

Carbohydrates

Although carbohydrates are not considered to be an essential nutrient, they are our body's main source of energy. They are comprised mostly of carbon (C), hydrogen (H), and oxygen (O) atoms. The body utilizes most carbohydrates to generate glucose, which serves as the basic functional particle of energy within the cells. Kilocalories (kcal) are the result, with an average of 4 kcal per gram (kcal/g) of carbohydrates. A kilocalorie is equivalent to one calorie on a nutritional label of a packaged food.[8] Not all carbohydrates are the same, however. Simple sugars are the smallest carbohydrates and are made up of one or two sugar molecules. Polysaccharides are complex carbohydrates and are made up of many sugar molecules. Some examples of these forms of carbohydrates are potatoes, beans, and vegetables. Dietary fiber is another form of complex carbohydrates where the sugar molecules are linked together. However, the body cannot usually break these links apart and they pass through with minimal changes.

Proteins

I am sure that we have all heard of the importance of protein. The emphasis is not exaggerated at all. Every cell in our body contains proteins. Protein is essential for tissue growth and cellular repair. It is also the major component in the makeup of bone, muscle, and other tissues and fluids. They are created through the process of linking different combinations and large quantities of the twenty amino acids or building blocks found in our food. Our inherited genes typically dictate how the proteins are formed. When used as an energy source, protein supplies an average of 4 kilocalories per gram. In the American diet today, it is rare to come across a case of protein deficiency. Most Americans eat up to two times the required protein portion necessary to maintain adequate health.

Fats & Lipids

Lipids consist of fats and oils. Fat is basically concentrated energy that yields high volumes of energy producing molecules. They are composed mostly of carbon (C), hydrogen (H) and oxygen (O). Fats and lipids are an important part of bodily function. They assist in helping our bodies to store fat-soluble vitamins and provide high levels of stored energy for when we need it. Fats are stored by the body in the form of fat tissue which also cushions and protects our internal organs and skeletal infrastructure. A healthy diet should consist of no more than thirty percent fat. Unfortunately, we are seeing that fat consumption is way above the recommended dosage in average people's diets, leading to detrimental states of health such as the obesity crisis and diabetes epidemic. Studies show that four out of five people with type 2 diabetes are overweight or obese. Excess fat, especially abdominal fat, changes the way that the body responds to insulin, leading to a condition called insulin resistance. With this condition, the cells cannot use insulin to process blood sugar out of the blood, resulting in high blood sugar levels.

Vitamins

There are thirteen essential vitamins that are required for the human body to function properly. Four of these vitamins can be produced in the body naturally but usually in insufficient amounts. With that being said, they must be provided for through dietary consumption. Otherwise, the body will experience the symptoms of deficiency for that particular nutrient. Vitamins are divided into two categories: **water-soluble** and **fat-soluble**. Vitamins A, D, E, and K are the four fat-soluble vitamins. The eight B vitamins and vitamin C make up the other nine water-soluble vitamins. Of the eight B vitamins, two are made in our intestines. Each vitamin contributes its own characteristics in the role of human and even animal health. Contrary to popular belief, avoiding fats completely can be harmful to the body. Fats do play an important role in fat-soluble vitamins' ability to be absorbed by the body. Fat-soluble vitamins are stored in the body's fatty tissue. They are absorbed more easily by the body in the presence of dietary fat. Because much of your body consists of water, many of the water-soluble vitamins circulate easily throughout the body. The kidneys continuously regulate their levels by discharging excesses out of the body in urine. They are absorbed directly into the bloodstream as food is broken down in the digestion process. Normally, water-soluble vitamins do not remain in the body for very long. Vitamin B12 is the only water-soluble vitamin that can be stored in the liver for many years.

Minerals

Trace minerals are exactly what they sound like. They are minerals where only traces are found in the human body. They are distinctly inorganic compounds with usually nothing more than a molecule or two of an element. Although minerals do not contribute to energy production, they support other vital functions that we require to survive. They promote cellular reactions, help to balance the water levels in the body and support structural systems, such as the skeletal system. Major minerals are more prevalent in the body; however, they are no more important to a person's health than trace minerals are. Major minerals travel through and enrich our bodies in different ways. For example, potassium behaves much like water-soluble vitamins do. It is quickly absorbed into the blood stream where it can circulate freely until it is excreted by the kidneys. In contrast, calcium requires a carrier for absorption and transport. Iron is an essential mineral critical for motor and cognitive development. When iron levels are low, a disease called anemia occurs. Iron deficiency is considered the most common and widespread nutritional disorder in the world according to the World Health Organization.[9] It is not only a significant crisis in developing countries but developed and industrialized countries as well.[8]

Food for Thought

There is no super-food that contains the full range of essential vitamins and minerals that a human needs in order to survive. However, there are plant-based foods that contain many of them. For example, Kale is known to be a nutrient powerhouse and scientists are discovering more and more health benefits that are derived from parts of the Moringa tree. The wonderful thing about eating diets that are plant-based is the fact that they have been known to prevent and even reverse the onset of chronic illnesses such as diabetes, cardiovascular disease, hypertension and more. They also contain no cholesterol and very few calories or fat. Many studies now report the potential health risk with diets high in red and processed meat, animal fats, processed foods, sugar, salts, and additives. Scientists also have confirmed that a diet high in fruits, vegetables, nuts, seeds and whole grains is essential to prevent and cure chronic diseases and some cancers.

Vegetables

Nutrient-dense green vegetables—leafy greens, cruciferous vegetables, and other green vegetables—are the most important foods to focus on in your diet. In fact, greens are the number one food you can eat regularly to help improve your health.

57

Medical professionals typically will recommend that a person eats five or more servings of vegetables per day. These types of foods are even known to aid in the prevention and reversal of diabetes. Higher green vegetable consumption is associated with a lower risk of developing type 2 diabetes, and among diabetics, higher green vegetable intake is associated with lower HbA1c levels. A recent meta-analysis found that greater leafy green intake was associated with a 14% decrease in risk of type 2 diabetes. One study reported that each daily serving of leafy greens produces a 9% decrease in risk of developing diabetes.

As mentioned previously, Kale is a powerhouse, nutrient rich food that is an excellent source of vitamins A, C, and K has a good amount of calcium for a vegetable, and also supplies folate and potassium. Other noteworthy greens include:

- Spinach
- Collard Greens
- Broccoli
- Romaine Lettuce

Non-starchy vegetables like mushrooms, onions, garlic, eggplant, and peppers are essential components of chronic illness prevention (or reversal) diet. These foods have almost non-existent effects on blood glucose and are packed with fiber and phytochemicals.

Fruits

Most fruits are naturally low in fat, sodium, and calories and, as with vegetables, none of them contain cholesterol. They are good sources of many essential nutrients that are under-consumed in our society today, including:

- potassium
- dietary fiber
- vitamin C
- and folate (folic acid)

Research shows that healthy potassium consumption in a person's diet may help to maintain healthy blood pressure. Dietary fiber obtained from fruits helps to reduce blood cholesterol levels and may even lower a person's risk of heart disease. Fiber is important for proper bowel function. It helps reduce constipation and diverticulosis. Fiber-containing foods such as fruits help provide a feeling of fullness with fewer calories. It is important to note, however, that although whole or cut-up fruits are great sources of dietary fiber, *fruit juices* may contain little or no fiber at all. Fruits are also great sources of Vitamin C, which is important for growth and repair of all body tissues, helps heal cuts and wounds, and keeps teeth and gums healthy. Folate (folic acid) helps the body form red blood cells. Women of childbearing age who may become pregnant should consume adequate folate from foods, and in addition 400 mcg of synthetic folic acid from fortified foods

59

or supplements. This reduces the risk of neural tube defects, spina bifida, and anencephaly during fetal development.

Nuts & Seeds

Nuts and seeds are natural hunger-busters, not only because of their fat content but also because of their protein and fiber content. All nuts contain fiber, which helps lower cholesterol while anchoring a person's blood sugar. Most nuts, especially peanuts, contain other slimming nutrients. Peanuts could be considered the unsung heroes when it comes to building lean muscle mass because they contain the non-essential amino acid L-arginine. It's being studied for its ability to lessen body fat while helping to build lean muscle mass at the same time. Nuts also contain a wide array of antioxidants and vital minerals that most people lack, like:

- Manganese
- Calcium
- Iron
- Chromium
- Zinc
- Selenium which is important for many physiological and metabolic functions.

If you're looking to lose fat, eating fats for weight loss is so important! It might seem counter-intuitive, but not getting enough good quality fats along with other vital nutrients in your diet can sabotage your weight loss efforts.

Grains

Healthcare practitioners recommend that people eat at least three or more servings of whole grains each day. Processed grains such as polished rice and white flour are stripped of their nutritional values and need to be artificially fortified with the necessary vitamins and minerals that the human body requires for good health. In fact, the disease beriberi was a direct result of stripping those nutrients from the rice during processing. *Whole grains*, on the other hand, such as:

- Brown rice
- Barley
- Rye
- Quinoa
- Bulgar wheat
- Whole wheat bread and pasta

...are packed with essential vitamins and minerals and are a great source of nutrients such as fiber, calcium, and others. Moreover, grains are essential because they offer great sources of good carbohydrates which the body uses as energy.

Beans, Lentils, and other legumes

Beans, lentils, and other legumes are the ideal carbohydrate source. Beans are low in GL due to their moderate protein and abundant fiber and resistant starch, carbohydrates that are not

61

broken down in the small intestine. This reduces the amount of calories that can be absorbed from beans. Additionally, resistant starch is fermented by bacteria in the colon, forming products that protect against colon cancer. Accordingly, bean and legume consumption is associated with reduced risk of both diabetes and colon cancer.

Beans are very high in fiber and low on the glycemic index. They give you about 1/3 of your daily fiber requirements in just a 1/2 cup (at around 190 calories) and are also good sources of magnesium (important for heart health) and potassium (crucial for muscle function and hydration). Like berries and greens, beans are in the running for the top anti-oxidant rich foods, a little-known fact. Kidney and red beans rank highest, then black beans following close behind. Black beans are especially good for digestive tract health and have been studied in the context of colon cancer. If you have trouble digesting beans, here are two easy tips:

- Start by eating small portions, say 2 heaping tablespoons, to help your digestion become used to them until they cause less discomfort.
- If you don't mind cooking your beans from scratch, soaking dried beans helps remove some of the flatulence-causing substances.

As with everything in life, it is important to remember the rule of **moderation**. Portion size is a substantial aspect of healthy eating habits. Unrealistic portion sizes are one of the top causes of over-eating. Today, modern packaging does not exemplify correct portion sizes for a healthy diet. A good example of an appropriate portion size is an amount equal to the size of a person's fist for most foods.

In Summary

In 1896, on his return to the Netherlands and after his discovery of the cause of the disease beriberi, Christiaan Eijkman declared that "White rice can be poisonous!" Gerrit Grinjs, who continued Eijkman's research at the institute after he left, did more research and understood that white rice wasn't toxic, but that it lacked something vital – its natural and proper nutritional value. By not fueling our bodies with foods that provide us the nutrition we need, we are creating hazardous conditions inside of our own selves. Fueling our bodies and making sure that we have all the nutrients that we need for proper functionality just cannot be neglected if we want to maximize our health and our quality of life.

Just about 99% of human body mass is made up of six collective elements. They are oxygen, carbon, hydrogen, nitrogen, calcium, and phosphorus. Another five elements, potassium, sulfur, sodium, chlorine, and magnesium make up the other 0.85%. Every single one of these elements is vital to life and we need to ensure that we do our part by giving our bodies what they need through healthy nutrition. Today many researchers have shown that the number one cause of poor health and death in the USA is related to our diet.

63

5

E- Exercise: Regular Physical Exercise is Medicine

On September 2, 2013, Diana Nyad became the first person to ever swim from Cuba to Key West, Florida, without using a shark cage. It was a record-setting swim that captured the hearts and the imagination of the world, not because Nyad swam that tremendous distance of one hundred and ten miles in just under fifty-three hours, enduring sun, tumultuous waves, illness, and jellyfish stings in the process, but because she was sixty-four years old when she did it. When she finally completed her historic swim on Monday, her first message was that you're never too old to chase your dreams. Nyad claims to be "in her prime" at sixty-four years of age, proving that you can exercise and be fit at any age. After all, age is just a number. At least that is what the world's oldest female bodybuilder Ernistine Shepard says. She began her fitness journey at age fifty-six. Now in her seventies, Shepard claims that she is in better shape than when she was in her forties.

Ernestine had lived her life as what she calls a "prissy" woman. She claimed to never have worked out a day in her life prior. You don't have to already be in shape in order to start exercising. You don't even need to have done it before. You can begin the journey of living an active and healthy life at anytime, anywhere and at any age. There is a famous saying that states "There is no time like the present." This couldn't be truer when it comes to health and fitness. Physical activity and exercise can benefit you throughout your life and, believe it or not, even your children's lives. Regular physical exercise is indeed medicine!

A Heritage of Risk Factors

Obesity has become a national crisis in recent years with approximately one in every three adults and one in every six children being overweight or obese. In fact, a new study by medical school researchers has shown that one of the major risk factors for children to become overweight or obese is having obese parents. According to the American Obesity Association, pediatricians are reporting more frequent cases of obesity-related diseases such as type-2 diabetes, asthma, and hypertension — diseases that once were previously considered adult conditions.[1] Obesity costs the United States over $200 billion and nearly twenty-one percent of the national medical budget each year.[2]

To put it in the simplest terms possible, obesity is a result of people consuming more calories each day than their bodies can burn; however, it is much more complicated than that. Over the past fifty years, there has been a shift in how Americans live and operate within their environments. Food has become more readily available and the opportunities for physical exercise are lacking. For example, technology and expansion have made it more difficult or even impractical to be physically active in some cases. Today, very few people will walk or ride a bicycle to their job or to drop their kids off at school because sometimes they work, or their children may go to school several miles away. Another example is that, in some less developed areas, walking, biking or jogging just isn't safe. There are still many areas and communities that do not have pedestrian friendly streets and roadways, making it difficult for people in those areas to get the physical exercise that they need. As technology advances, people are finding themselves sitting behind desks and staring at screens rather than doing any kind of physical exercise for work. Instead of playing outside, children are watching more and more television and playing video games.

Physical activity and exercise are crucial for a child's development. Research studies have observed a link between regular physical exercise and cognitive ability. In fact, in 2006, the *California Journal of Health Promotion* identified and published their findings of an association between physical education and academic achievement. The publication cited a study by California State University researchers that did a comparison of the difference between schools that had a fitness program and those that did not. When the students' test scores were reviewed, it was found out that the leading schools also had a structured physical education program based on the State Board of Education guidelines. On the other hand, the schools that had the lowest academic scores did not have any kind of physical education program, much less one that met any guidelines.[3]

An academic setting is but one arena where regular exercise can benefit the public. As adults, cognitive boosts could improve our performance at work. Some of the most noticeable benefits of physical exercise are our mental alertness and moods. When we exercise, our bodies release endorphins which boost mood, but we are also increasing blood flow to the brain, which can help sharpen our awareness and make us more ready to tackle our next big project. Engaging in physical exercise also gives us more energy throughout the day because it is a catalyst for the metabolic process. This helps us to feel more awake at work, even without caffeinated drinks such as coffee and tea, which can actually be harmful to the body. One of the most common excuses for not exercising is a lack of time. Many of us have busy lives with kids and work or even continuing education. Some people are single parents and have to raise a family alone. It is understandable to be strapped for time; however, there are small changes that you can make in your daily life and on a regular basis to meet your daily goals, such as walking during your lunch period or taking the stairs instead of the elevator.[5]

Lack of Physical Exercise and the Connection to Disease

Although exercise and physical activity are not the same, both can help to promote a healthy lifestyle. A sedentary lifestyle can lead to several different types of illnesses and disease. But what is the difference between physical activity and exercise? Medical and health researchers have focused on exercise, as well as on the more broadly defined concept of physical activity. Exercise is defined as a type of physical activity that is planned out and structured in such a way so as to be performed with the goal of improving health or fitness and then repeated. Studies on physical exercise in many groups, including men and women, children, teens, adults, older adults, people with disabilities, and women during pregnancy and the postpartum period, have focused on the role that physical activity plays in many health outcomes.

According to the American Diabetes Association, diabetes claims the lives of more people each year than breast cancer and AIDS combined. Although it is not the only risk factor contributing to diabetes, four out of five people with type 2 diabetes are overweight or obese. As I have mentioned previously, 80% of people that are diagnosed with type 2 diabetes have insulin resistance. This is a condition in which the insulin becomes ineffective in transporting blood sugar into the cells. This then promotes an unusually high level of glucose in the blood stream which consequently leads to pre-diabetes and subsequently type 2 diabetes.[4] John Thyfault, an assistant

69

professor in MU's departments of Nutrition and Exercise Physiology and Internal Medicine, has found that a lack of regular physical exercise impairs glycemic control, control of blood sugar levels, suggesting that inactivity may play a key role in the development of type 2 diabetes.[6]

Diabetes is only one of the many illnesses that can occur as a result of excess weight gain. Being overweight is also a risk factor in several types of cancer including breast cancer in women past menopause, colon and rectum cancer, endometrium cancer, which is a cancer of the lining of the uterus, and cancer of the esophagus, pancreas, and kidney, among several others. Being overweight can increase cancer risk in many ways. One of the main ways is that excess weight causes the body to produce and circulate more estrogen and insulin, hormones that can stimulate cancer growth.[7]

Exercise, Not Just Diet

Although dieting can shrink fat cells, it does not completely eliminate them, which is why people can gain the weight back so quickly. Regular physical exercise creates a metabolic pattern that is absolutely crucial to a healthy lifestyle. In fact, aside from quitting smoking, *or not smoking at all*, exercise is probably one of the most powerful lifestyle choices that a person can make in order to improve their health. Maintaining a healthy exercise regimen for your weight, gender and age will help the body to burn the calories that you eat instead of starving yourself and binge eating later on down the road.

Obviously, when you exercise, your body burns calories to fuel your activity, but exercise is the gift that keeps on giving. Even after your workout has ended, your body is still burning calories during the metabolic process because muscle itself burns calories even when you are in a state of rest.

Christopher Wharton, PhD, a certified personal trainer and researcher with the Rudd Center for Food Policy and Obesity at Yale University, says that a person's metabolic rate, which is a measurement of the amount of calories burned per day in adults, can be elevated as a result of aerobic exercise for at least twenty-four hours. It is hard to pinpoint exactly how long this effect lasts for each individual because there are several different contributing factors that play a role, such as body composition and a person's level of training. If you want to prolong this calorie-burning effect, Wharton advises exercising for longer periods.[8]

Strength, Aerobic and Flexibility Training For All Ages

Not only is physical exercise a great way to burn and reduce fat and prevent associated illnesses such as cancer and diabetes, but regular physical exercise can also help to strengthen muscles. Not just skeletal muscles though, but muscles such as the heart, and even your bones. There are many different forms of physical exercise. A few examples include:

- Strength training

- Aerobic training
- Flexibility training

Each one of these forms of exercise has its benefits for the human body. Unfortunately, there are some misconceptions about strength training.

Strength training, also known as resistance training, weight training, or muscle-strengthening activity, is one of the most beneficial components of a fitness program. Some people believe that if you lift weights or become very strong, you will automatically "bulk up" or gain more body mass. Women especially avoid this type of exercise for fear of gaining too much muscle mass. However, that is not how it works. When we strength train, our muscles do become stronger, therefore increasing our muscle and in effect, our body mass. However, studies have shown that strength training increases _lean_ body mass, decreases fat mass, and increases the body's resting metabolic rate. While strength training on its own typically does not lead to weight loss, its beneficial effects on body composition may make it easier to manage one's weight and ultimately reduce the risk of disease, by slowing the gain of fat — especially abdominal fat. Muscle is metabolically active tissue. It utilizes calories to work, repair, and refuel itself. Fat, on the other hand, doesn't use as much energy.[9]

Part of the natural aging process includes a slow reduction in muscle. That means that our bodies require fewer calories each day. If we continue in the same eating patterns into older adulthood, we might be consuming more calories than we need every day and it becomes easier to gain weight. Strength training regularly helps preserve our lean muscle tissue and can even rebuild some that have been lost already. Weight training has also been shown to help fight osteoporosis. For example, a study in postmenopausal women examined whether regular strength training and high-impact aerobics sessions would help prevent osteoporosis. Researchers found that the women who participated in at least two sessions a week for three years were able to preserve bone mineral density at the spine and hip. Over the same time period, a sedentary control group showed bone mineral density losses of 2 to 8 percent.[10]

In older populations, resistance training can help maintain the ability to perform functional tasks such as walking, rising from a chair, climbing stairs, and even carrying one's own groceries. A systematic review of 8 studies examining the effects of weight-bearing and resistance-based exercises on the bone mineral density (BMD) in older men found resistance training to be an effective strategy for preventing osteoporosis in this population. Resistance training was found to have more positive effects on BMD than walking, which has a lower impact.

The Exercise Guidelines for Americans recommends that muscle strengthening activities be done at least two days a week. Different types of strength training activities are best for different age groups. When talking about the benefits of exercise, keeping the heart and blood vessels healthy usually gets most of the attention. For many individuals, though, stretching and strength training exercises may be just as important.

Flexibility training or stretching exercise is another important part of overall fitness. It may help older adults preserve the range of motion they need to perform daily tasks and other physical activities. The American Heart Association recommends that healthy adults engage in flexibility training two to three days per week, stretching major muscle and tendon groups. For older adults, the American Heart Association and American College of Sports Medicine recommend two days a week of flexibility training, in sessions at least 10 minutes long. Older adults who are at risk of falling should also do exercises to improve their balance.[11]

During **aerobic activity**, you repeatedly move large muscles in your arms, legs and hips. The breathing rate becomes faster and deeper which maximizes the amount of oxygen in the blood. The heart rate increases and rapidly pumps the blood to the muscles and back to the lungs. The small blood vessels, called capillaries, will widen to deliver more oxygen to your muscles and carry away waste products, such as carbon dioxide and lactic acid. Our bodies even release endorphins which are natural painkillers that promote an increased sense of well-being. Over time and with regular practice, aerobic exercises can increase overall cardiovascular health on a long term scale by increasing the body's efficiency of respiration, improving the blood volume, and increasing blood distribution and delivery to the muscles.

According to the Centers for Disease Control and Prevention, additional health benefits of physical exercise include:

- **Control your weight**
- **Reduce your risk of cardiovascular disease**
- **Reduce your risk for type 2 diabetes and metabolic syndrome**
- **Reduce your risk of some cancers**
- **Strengthen your bones and muscles**
- **Improve your mental health and mood**
- **Improve your ability to do daily activities and prevent falls, if you're an older adult**
- **Increase your chances of living longer**

How Many Calories Are You Burning?

Although there are several health benefits of exercise and physical activity, one of the main reasons why people exercise is because they either want to lose weight or stay fit and healthy. Caloric intake and expenditure play a big role in both of those scenarios. When people exercise, they typically want to know how many calories they are burning as they exercise. We briefly touched on metabolic rate earlier but now we are going to go a bit more in-depth into the subject. As we mentioned before, a person's metabolic rate determines how many calories that person's body will burn while they are at rest. The more lean muscle mass a person has, the more calories their body will burn. There is a simple formula that you can use to help you determine what your BMR is or your basic metabolic rate, and it is different respectively for males and females. A few key factors that need to be determined before you can begin the figuring process, however, are your height, weight, and age. Once you have these three things, you can just plug the numbers right into the formula to discover just what your metabolic rate is.

Weight = W
Height = H
Age = A

- **Men**: BMR = 66.47 + (13.75 x W) + (5.0 x H) - (6.75 x A)
- **Women**: BMR = 665.09 + (9.56 x W) + (1.84 x H) - (4.67 x A)

There are several different ways that you can calculate how many calories you burn for the various exercises based off of your BMR, but it is important to remember to factor in the amount of calories that your body requires each day at rest to satisfy daily demands. As a basic rule of thumb, the human body will require about 60% of daily consumed calories each day for normal bodily function. The other 40% is used for physical exercise and digestion (digestion only constituting about 10% of that).

Of course, if you don't want to do all the math, there are calculators that you can use where you just punch in the details as far as age, height, weight and activity and they will give you your customized results. However, for some of the most common activities, the calculations have already been done. From a simple walk to a brisk run and even general gardening can burn calories. So no matter what your physical exercise of preference is, you can live a healthy and fit lifestyle by doing just about anything.

Intensity: Recommendations

Intensity is another important aspect of physical exercise that many people do not account for. This is primarily because not everyone's intensity levels are the same. There are basically three different levels of intensity. They are:

- **Low**
- **Moderate**
- **High**

Just because a workout or physical exercise seems simple to some, that does not mean that it couldn't be a high-intensity workout to others. Take walking for example. For a person who is in great shape and runs marathons, of course, walking would be literally "a walk in the park." For others who may be obese or live a primarily sedentary lifestyle, walking half a mile could be a nearly impossible feat. So instead of categorizing intensity levels by the type of physical exercise that it is, we are going to cover intensity by the results that they produce and their characteristics. The intensity of a physical exercise is based upon how that person feels during and after the workout. Breathing and heart rate are huge factors that should be considered. Other factors include sweating and muscle fatigue.

Low: Obviously, a low-intensity physical exercise is a workout where the individual performing the actions feels few effects as a result of elevated breathing and heart rate. They may not sweat and should experience no muscle fatigue or soreness.

Moderate: Moderate activities are those that make you breathe a little harder and your heart rate should be slightly more elevated. After extended periods of moderate physical exercise, you may feel some muscle fatigue. A person could break a sweat during activities at this intensity, but it is not a strong determining factor.

High: Vigorous activities make you use large muscle groups and make your heart beat considerably faster. Respiration is dramatically increased and, a majority of the time, vigorous physical exercise will also make you sweat.

So how much physical exercise do you need each week to ensure that you are doing the best for your body? The latest recommendations for adults and older adults calls for at least 150 minutes of moderate intensity or 75 minutes of vigorous intensity activity each week, or an equivalent combination, preferably spread throughout the week. This is over and above usual daily activities like using the stairs instead of the elevator at your office or doing house or yard work. For children, the recommendation is at least 60 minutes of moderate or vigorous intensity activity each day, with vigorous intensity activity occurring at least 3 days each week. It's important to limit sedentary behavior such as sitting, lying down, watching television, or other forms of screen-based entertainment.[12]

If you currently don't exercise and aren't very active during the day, any increase in physical exercise is good for you. Some studies show that walking briskly for even one to two hours a week (15 to 20 minutes a day) starts to decrease the chances of having a heart attack or stroke, developing diabetes, or dying prematurely.

In Summary

Children and adolescents should get at least 1 hour or more a day of physical exercise in age-appropriate activities, spending most of that engaged in moderate- or vigorous–intensity aerobic activities. They should partake in vigorous-intensity aerobic activity on at least three days of the week and include muscle strengthening and bone strengthening activities on at least three days of the week.

Healthy adults should get a minimum of 2-1/2 hours per week of moderate-intensity aerobic activity, or a minimum of 1-1/4 hours per week of vigorous-intensity aerobic activity, or a combination of the two. That could mean a brisk walk for 30 minutes a day, five days a week; a high-intensity spinning class one day for 45 minutes, plus a half hour jog another day; or some other combination of moderate and vigorous activity. Doubling the amount of activity (5 hours moderate- or 2-1/2 hours of vigorous-intensity aerobic activity) provides even more health benefits. Adults should also aim to do muscle-strengthening activities at least two days a week.

Healthy older Adults should follow the guidelines for healthy adults. Older adults who cannot meet the guidelines for healthy adults because of chronic conditions should be as physically active as their abilities and conditions allow. People who have chronic conditions such as arthritis and type 2 diabetes should talk to a healthcare provider about the amount and type of activity that is best. Physical exercise can help people manage chronic conditions, as long as the activities that individuals choose match their fitness level and abilities. Even just an hour a week of activity has health benefits. Older adults who are at risk of falling should include activities that promote balance.[13]

Although there is no one, simple solution to the obesity crisis and the steady decrease in physical exercise, there are steps that can be taken in order to help them. It will require the efforts of the combined communities and not just the individuals because safety must be a priority when being active or promoting active lifestyles. Roadways and streets need to offer safe places to cross for pedestrians and cyclists, sidewalks should be provided and cleaned where people can get from place to place on foot and parks and nature trails should be well lit and patrolled to ensure that people are protected while out exercising.

6

A=Access to Healthcare Screening

A Tale of Two Patients

B reast cancer is one of the leading causes of death among women in the United States and other parts of the world. (One in eight women will develop breast cancer during her lifetime.) Over the last twenty-five years of my practice, I've seen many patients with this disease. Some are still alive today while, unfortunately, others have not had the same fate. Although disease prevention is ideal, early detection is the next best option. When diseases are detected early, then the patient has the ability to respond more favorably to the treatment of choice because the earlier a disease is diagnosed, the more likely it is that it can be cured or successfully managed.

Several years ago, a patient of mine, a healthcare provider, came to me with the complaint of a lump in her breast. I quickly assessed the patient and then ordered a series of tests to clearly define the nature of this breast lump. After the mammogram was completed, a mass was confirmed. In most cases, patients with complaints such as an unusual swelling or growth will be recommended by their primary care physician to have specific health screenings, to fully determine the cause of such abnormality. In this particular case, a mammogram and a breast sonogram were the tests of choice. After reviewing the mammogram result with the patient, I immediately sent her to the surgeon for evaluation and a subsequent breast biopsy. The results of the biopsy showed that the mass was indeed a cancerous tumor.

As soon as the lump was confirmed to be cancer, the patient was quickly referred to the appropriate subspecialty doctors for treatment. She responded well to treatment and remained cancer free for many years. Surprisingly enough a few years ago this same patient returned again with the same complaint of a lump, but this time in the other breast. We followed the same diagnostic pathway and the patient had her mastectomy and was doing well. Then one day she came to me complaining that she just did not feel right – as if something was wrong but she couldn't tell what it could be. She was getting tired easily although she did not have any significant pain nor was she necessarily losing weight. However, given her history of bilateral breast cancer, I decided to order what is called a metastatic workup for her. This screening is designed to look for certain types of cancers such as breast cancer that may have spread to other parts of the body such as the lungs, liver or kidneys. Unfortunately, we found a tumor in one of her kidneys that was also malignant. With a sense of urgency, we worked to get her treated. Finally, the patient had the kidney removed and she is now doing very well. Having access to healthcare is very important. Without access to healthcare, this patient's story would probably be very different.

Typically, initial mammograms are done at age forty unless a patient displays symptoms that suggest that a mammogram be done earlier. For example, I had another patient who was in her thirties who came to me with the complaint of a lump in her breast that had grown exponentially over the last several weeks. When I examined the patient, I realized that things were not looking good for her at all. A mammogram and a sonogram were ordered immediately and these tests confirmed that she did indeed have a mass that had all the characteristics of malignancy. She was then referred to surgery and had her mastectomy done but it was already late. The cancer had spread to many of her internal organs. The cancer had now gone from an early stage, where the disease would have been more manageable, to an advanced stage. The treatment was not effective because the cancer was not detected in time. The patient suffered. She endured much pain despite appropriate pain management until we eventually lost her. This story is to emphasize that disease prevention is the gold standard, but the next best thing is early detection.

Finding and Treating Diseases at an Early Stage Can Save Lives

There are many reasons why diseases such as cancer and Alzheimer's can be detected late. One of the most common reasons is that people often do not know what to look for or some of the common signs and symptoms associated with the disease. Unfortunately, around 1 in 4 of cancers is diagnosed through emergency admission to hospital. Most of the patients diagnosed in this way usually do not have favorable outcomes and their chances of survival are extremely low. Another reason why detection may be late is that sometimes, patients are afraid to confirm their fears. They oftentimes do not want to hear that they have cancer or Alzheimer's disease or diabetes. These illnesses are life-threatening and a diagnosis can be terrifying. Some people may not know how to handle the news or how to cope with those kinds of grim circumstances.

Although it may be a scary scenario to face, early detection and diagnosis save lives. In fact, studies show that in both breast and ovarian cancer, more than 90% of women diagnosed at the earliest stages survive their disease for at least 5 years compared to around 15% for women diagnosed with the most advanced stage of breast cancer or around 5% for women diagnosed with the most advanced stage of ovarian cancer. Even 70% of lung cancer patients will survive for at least a year if diagnosed at the earliest stage compared to around 14% for people diagnosed with the most advanced stage of disease.[1]

For cognitive degenerative diseases, early detection can help in many ways. For example:

1. Catching the disease at a stage when it could still be reversed: even if there is an underlying dementia such as Alzheimer's disease, diagnosis, and treatment of reversible conditions can help to improve brain function and reduce symptoms.

2. The disease may still be treatable and treatment could result in a full recovery or at least greatly reduce the chances of further decline.

3. Early diagnoses are also more accurate because the patient might still be able to answer key questions or report concerns that others may not notice. These kinds of results are more difficult to achieve when a large part of the brain has become affected.

4. It will allow the patient to participate more in the preparation of short-term and long-term care and planning such as legal and financial matters as well as being able to make their wishes known to their family members.

5. It will also allow the patient the opportunity to reprioritize how they spend their time so that they can enjoy and make the most of it such as spending time with family and friends, traveling or creating a deeper spiritual connection with God.

6. An early diagnosis will also help the family to prepare for the disease through education. Educating your

family members about the disease will help to reduce their stress as well as feelings of regret and remorse.

Individuals diagnosed early in the disease process can take advantage of support groups in the early stages and learn tips and strategies from others in similar situations to better manage and cope with their symptoms. New research and technology are emerging every day and there are clinical trials that help to further the development of treatments to improve the care of patients suffering from disease and increase their opportunities. Advocacy groups also help others to understand more about diseases and the stigmas associated with them. For example, mental changes in a person who has some kind of cognitive degenerative disease can attribute those changes to the disease rather than to their own personal failings. Altogether, these advantages result in a higher quality of life for the person afflicted, less stress for family care partners, and more time to treasure the present and prepare for the future.[2]

The Unfortunate Truth

In 2010, the U.S. Department of Health & Human Services Centers for Disease Control and Prevention reported that seven of the top ten causes of death in the United States were the result of chronic diseases. Heart disease and cancer alone accounted for nearly 48% of all of those deaths. In 2012, the American Diabetes Association did a study that confirmed that approximately 29 million people in the United States have diabetes. That is 9.3% of the national population. Of that 29 million, 8.1 million were undiagnosed.[3] Diabetes is the leading cause of kidney failure, lower-limb amputations other than those caused by injury, and new cases of blindness among Americans today. Worldwide, there are about 300 million diabetics and that number is continuously rising. If present trends continue, experts believe that diabetes will afflict nearly 1 in every 3 people in their lifetime. So when you think about just how many people might actually have diabetes and don't know about it, it is quite alarming. Nearly 27.8% of people living with diabetes don't even know that they have it and therefore are not treating it. If left untreated and without the proper access to healthcare, diabetes can ultimately lead to untimely death and/or a poor quality of life.

The Biggest Killer

Physicians and medical experts are becoming increasingly alarmed at the rate of people who are dying from hypertension-related deaths such as heart failure or kidney failure. In 2015, a new report was released by the American Heart Association that confirmed that deaths caused by high blood pressure were on the rise. High blood pressure is one of the greatest risk factors for a wide variety of serious and potentially life-threatening medical complications, and cardiovascular disease is still considered one of the biggest killers in the United States. Approximately 80 million Americans are afflicted with high blood pressure and only about half of those people have the condition under control. In fact, some experts believe that there are populations suffering from hypertension that go undertreated. Awareness campaigns and community-based initiatives help more and more people to control their blood pressure successfully, but these measures are oftentimes not enough. However, as healthcare systems around the country better implement evidence-based prevention and treatment guidelines from the AHA and the American College of Cardiology, a slight decrease in the number of American deaths attributed to heart disease and stroke was reported according to new statistics from the American Heart Association.[4]

The Importance of Health Screenings

Early detection and having an adequate level of access to healthcare can increase a person's longevity and quality of life. It is vital that patients report any changes or concerns that they are experiencing to their primary care physicians as soon as they appear. Because most patients have not had medical training of any kind, it is common that, although they may be experiencing symptoms of chronic illness, they may not be able to identify them as the first signs of a potential health problem. This is why regular health screenings are so crucial. They are intended to identify health concerns before they develop any further and therefore increase the patient's chance of a successful treatment plan and possible full remission of the disease.

Health screenings such as mammograms, pap smears, and colorectal tests can find cancer at its early stages when the diseases are easier to treat and the patients will be more receptive to the treatment. The different types of health screenings will mostly be recommended for a patient dependent upon that person's age unless they are showing signs that a screening should be performed earlier.

- Breast Cancer Screenings (Mammograms) – Women ages 40 and above should get yearly mammograms to test for breast cancer.
- Colon and rectal cancer and polyps – Both men and women should begin these health screenings starting at age 50 and above. Physicians also recommend:
  a) Flexible sigmoidoscopy every 5 years
  b) Colonoscopy every 10 years
  c) Double-contrast barium enema every 5 years
  d) CT colonography (virtual colonoscopy) every 5 years
- Cervical cancer screenings (Pap smears) – This health screening is not recommended for women under the age of 21 unless they are showing signs that a screening should be performed earlier. However, from age 21 to 29 a Pap test should be done at least once every three years. HPV testing is usually not conducted unless the patient has an abnormal pap smear. Between the ages of 30 and 65, however, both the Pap smear and HPV test should be done. If a woman has had her uterus and cervix removed (a hysterectomy) for reasons other

than cervical cancer, these types of screenings need not be completed.

- Prostate Cancer – The American Cancer Society recommends that men ages 50 and above be screened for prostate cancer, or younger if they have a family history of the disease.

- Blood Pressure – Both men and women ages 20 or over should be tested at least once every two years for high blood pressure. Typically, high blood pressure symptoms go unnoticed which makes this disease increasingly dangerous. Screenings are the best way to determine, treat and potentially reverse high blood pressure.

- Blood Glucose – At age 45 and above, both men and women should have their blood glucose levels tested by their primary care physician at least once every three years unless there is an indication that the screening be done earlier.

- Cholesterol (fasting lipoprotein profile) – Beginning at age 20, the fasting lipoprotein profile should be conducted at least once every 4-6 years for people of "normal risk." High-risk individuals should see their primary care physicians about regular screenings, especially if they have a family history of the disease. High cholesterol elevates a person's risk for heart disease and stroke.

Of course, a person's health history is a great influencer of the needs of each individual patient. A primary care physician should always be consulted for the best course of action.[5]

The Golden Standard

Early detection greatly increases a person's receptiveness to treatments of several different diseases and chronic illnesses; however, disease prevention is the "Golden Standard" that every person should strive to achieve. There are several ways that you can help to prevent disease and chronic illness in your own life through lifestyle choices that you make. Getting regular and seasonal immunizations for some of the most common illnesses will not only help you to avoid illnesses in the first place, but will also prevent the spread of diseases as well. Different types of vaccines will help your body defend against full-blown viruses that in the past may have been life-threatening such as smallpox, polio, rabies and the flu. Reducing your risk factors is another one of the biggest steps that you can take toward living a longer and healthier lifestyle. Some of the ways that you can reduce your risk factors for cancer and other chronic illnesses and diseases are:

- Stay away from all forms of tobacco.
- Maintain a healthy weight for your age, gender and body type.
- Engage in regular physical activity.
- Eat a healthy plant-based diet.

- Avoid drinking alcohol.
- Protect your skin.
- Know yourself, your family history, and your risks.
- Get regular check-ups, immunizations and cancer screening tests.
- Find spiritual renewal and reduce your stress levels.

In Summary

The "access to healthcare" situation in the United States has been unreliable at best for several years. However, in 2014, 32 million Americans flooded the medical healthcare system with the passing of the Affordable Care Act. Unfortunately, this measure did not solve the problem and millions are still either not insured at all or are under-insured. The Office of Disease Prevention and Health Promotion announced that its goal for 2020 was to improve the American people's access to comprehensive and quality health care services.[7] Many times, people do not get the access to healthcare services that they need because either there is a lack of availability, the cost is too high or there is a lack of insurance coverage. These three major factors contribute to barriers in society's health needs creating more problems in the long run. Patients will experience delays in receiving the appropriate care and have the inability to attain preventative services such as healthcare screenings or immunizations and vaccines. Countless hospitalizations across the country could be totally prevented if people's access to healthcare services was greater, saving the national medical budget millions of dollars annually.

Achieving the best health outcomes is possible if everyone takes action and does their part. As individuals, we need to take responsibility for our actions and strive to reduce our own risk factors by living and eating healthier and staying active and fit. As a community, we need to come together to ensure that people have regular and ongoing sources of care, such as annual Mega Clinics, to increase health outcomes and reduce disparities and costs. By providing these simple health care services, we can prevent illness and the spread of diseases and viruses by detecting early warning signs and immunizing before they ever even begin, resulting in healthier communities across the nation and around the world.

L = Liquid: Adequate Consumption of Water Will Treat or Cure Most Diseases

When the earth was first formed, it was created in such a way that water was one of the most abundant resources on the planet. It was designed in this manner because of the critical role that water plays in all life on earth. Wherever water is found, you can be sure that life can be found there as well. Even in the most hostile and arid environments, scientists have discovered microbes, invertebrates and other life forms that have found a way to survive as long as there is some form of water. Just so you have an idea of how important water is to life on this planet, here is an analogy. Approximately thirty-one percent of the earth's surface is covered in forests that account for the world's oxygen supply — seventy-one percent is covered in water.[1] Now consider what sustains those mighty forests. What is the most important element to their survival?

Water. So either directly or indirectly, water is possibly the most important component for our continued existence.

About ninety-six percent of our water is in our oceans. Rivers, lakes, and glaciers are obvious water sources also, but what many people tend to forget is that water is all around us as water vapor in the air, in the soil as moisture, groundwater, and aquifers and even in every last cell in our bodies. Water is life's most basic necessity and without it, all living things on this planet would perish. It is in everything that we do, from physical activity and digestion to brain function and sleep. Nothing we do is possible without water.

In this book, I have discussed several key essentials that our bodies need in order to be healthy. I have gone over exercise and physical activity and the role that it plays in longevity. I went over different dietary necessities that the body requires for health including:

- Good carbohydrates
- Plant-based protein
- Fiber
- Vitamins and minerals
- Even good, plant-based fats

However, taking in all those other essential nutrients will not sustain us without water's help. In fact, under extreme circumstances of survival, a healthy human adult can survive nearly a month without any food, but only a few days without water.[2]

The Role of Water in our Bodies

It is common knowledge that our bodies are composed of anywhere between sixty and seventy-five percent water. With that being said, it is no wonder that almost every cell in our bodies depends on water. Water carries nutrients to our cells and helps us flush out toxins from our internal organs. Drinking water restores fluids that we lose through the processes of metabolism, our breathing, when we sweat and when our bodies remove waste. Yes, all of these bodily functions require water in order to complete their tasks, but it doesn't end there. Even if it is in small amounts, our bodies use water for a variety of other purposes such as:

- Regulating body temperature
- Moistening tissues in the eyes, mouth, throat, and nose
- Lubricating joints
- Protecting body organs and tissues
- Assisting in digestion
- Reducing stress on kidneys and liver by flushing out toxins
- Dissolving nutrients and allowing them to be absorbed by the body
- And so much more.
- May reduce the risk of acute heart attack

The importance of properly hydrating cannot be overstressed. It is highly recommended that you drink water before you begin to feel thirsty. That is because thirst is the first symptom of dehydration.[3] More than likely, if you are feeling thirsty, you are already dehydrated. During the hotter months of the year or when participating in any kind of physical activity, the amount of water that your bodies need increases with the level of activity that you are performing. The more rigorous the activity, or the hotter your environment, the more water you need to consume to stay sufficiently hydrated. Approximately twenty percent of our water comes from the foods we eat whereas eighty percent of our daily water intake comes from direct water consumption. That is why healthcare professionals stress the importance of drinking pure water.

Although there is water content in other drinks besides water, drinking pure water directly is the best way to hydrate. Other drinks such as sodas and caffeinated or sugary drinks contain high amounts of processed sugars, preservatives, caffeine and other ingredients that can actually be harmful to the body and can even dehydrate a person more. What many people fail to realize is that the body has to work harder to process and digest sugary and caffeinated drinks. Because water is used in the digestion process, the amount of water that it takes to break down all those extra refined and processed sugars and other toxins is more water than what the drink actually provides. In addition, those toxins need to also be excreted from the body and kidneys which require even more water usage.

Our Bodies Without Water

Did you know that most people are chronically dehydrated? Many of us may have become desensitized to the term "dehydration"; however, it is a very real threat that can even cost people their lives if not treated properly at its first signs. Did you know that more accidents occur during the warm weather months than any other time of year? As people head outdoors to enjoy what summer has to offer, they're not always the most careful and heat-related illnesses are a primary cause of this spike in hospitalizations. Long after their water bottles have gone dry, people are still out in the heat expending vast amounts of energy and sweat. When a person fails to replenish those liquids that they are losing, they become dehydrated.[4] That is why it is so critical to remember not only to hydrate properly but also what warning signs to look out for in case you or a loved one does become a victim of a heat-related illness.

Heat-related Illness

Lengthy or intense exposure to hot temperatures can cause heat-related illnesses. However, by reducing excessive exposure to high temperatures and taking other precautionary steps, most heat-related illnesses can be avoided. In fact, most people recover completely from heat-related illnesses if they are detected and treated early. On the other hand, if they are ignored, the consequences can be fatal.

Some examples of heat-related illnesses are:

- **Heat cramps**: Heat cramps are painful cramps that occur in the abdominal, leg and arm muscles as a result of a lack of fluids. They can strike when the body loses excessive amounts of fluids and salt.
- **Heat exhaustion**: Heat exhaustion is due to the loss of water and salt from heavy sweating. Signs include headache, nausea, dizziness, weakness, irritability, thirst, and heavy sweating. The person's pulse will be fast but weak. The skin will usually appear to be pale and may feel cold and clammy to the touch. It is not uncommon for a person to faint during heat exhaustion.
- **Heat stroke**: (also known as sun stroke) This is the most serious form of a heat-related illness on this list. If not detected or treated early, a person can end up suffering permanent damage or death from heatstroke. Most of the time, the signs and symptoms of heat cramps and heat exhaustion will have already occurred, so it is important not to ignore them and to seek treatment immediately. The person's body temperature will typically be above 103 degrees Fahrenheit, their skin will be hot and red, the pulse will be rapid and strong and the person may lose consciousness.

If you or someone you know is experiencing any of these signs and symptoms, it is crucial that you respond appropriately.

It could make the difference between life and death – literally. If the signs and symptoms are of heat exhaustion or heat cramps, move the person to a cooler location, loosen their clothing and try to cool the body with wet cloths or fanning. If the person is experiencing a heat or sun stroke, call 911 immediately. This is a medical emergency. Move the person to a cooler environment, try to reduce the person's body temperature by any means but DO NOT give the person fluids at this stage as it could cause medical complications.[5]

Water for Health, Healing & Hygiene

Water consumption is not the only way that water benefits us. It is also a key aspect of healing and hygiene which helps to keep us healthy as well. Let me give you an example. Puerperal infection, or childbed fever, is a devastating and life-threatening disease whose symptoms are very painful and prolonged. During the mid-1800s, this infection was prevalent among women who had just given birth – hence the adopted nickname "childbed fever." A puerperal infection, or puerperal sepsis, is a condition that occurs when a new mom experiences an infection related to giving birth.[6] Puerperal infections are the sixth-leading cause of death among new mothers, according to the World Health Organization (WHO).[7] For years, no one knew the cause of this disease until one day, a man by the name of Dr. Ignaz Semmelweis connected the practice of hand-washing to a reduction in the deaths of new mothers in Vienna.[8] Ever since then, hand-washing has revolutionized the

101

medical practice and has saved countless lives. Once people realized the importance of hand-washing, it became common practice in most developed societies around the world today and has helped prevent the spread of disease, germs, and infections for hundreds of years.

Hand-washing is only one way that water keeps us healthy. We use water to shower and bathe, cook and clean our food and so much more, but water also has healing properties that have been used for generations to heal a variety of ailments. The use of water for various treatments is probably as old as mankind, dating as far back as the ancient Greeks and Romans. The use of liquids as a treatment for medicinal purposes forms an integral part in many traditional medicine systems. Hydrotherapy, in general, includes several types of techniques in which water is used to heal the body. Hydrotherapy can be used as an internal treatment or an external treatment. External treatments are some of the most popular and they include showers and baths, neutral baths, sitz baths, contrasting foot and body baths, cold mitten friction rubs, steam inhalation for sinuses and congestion, alternating hot and cold compresses, heating compresses, body wraps and wet sheet packs.[9]

Water is also used externally to clean cuts and open sores, cool and reduce bruising, ease inflammation and even alleviate insect or animal bites. Hydrotherapy is commonly used for people suffering from arthritis and joint pain. In fact, aquatic exercises are commonly recommended for senior citizens in order to increase range of motion and promote healthy muscle maintenance without high impact stress on the muscles and joints. Hydro-massages are another great way that water is used to treat and heal the body. These specialized types of massages can be used to alleviate muscle or joint injuries as well as for stress and anxiety.

In Summary

So far I have gone over all the different aspects of water and how deeply it affects all of our lives, both directly and indirectly. We have stressed the importance of drinking plenty of water to keep our bodies hydrated, but what about the opposite – "over-hydrating"? You have probably heard stories of marathon runners and other athletes over-hydrating and drinking too much water. However, instances such as these are pretty uncommon. Not hydrating enough could lead to poor health. One question that is repeatedly asked is just how much water should a person drink each day. Eight glasses of water each day has traditionally been used as a rule of thumb; however, eight is not set in stone because there is no scientific evidence behind it according to Lynn Goldstein, a registered dietitian for HealthiNation.

There are several other factors that people need to consider when it comes to water consumption. Yes, recommendations vary between roughly eight to fifteen eight-ounce glasses of water each day but each individual is different. Size, activity levels, how hot it is outside, or how much heat exposure you get each day will all contribute to how much water is recommended for you specifically. People who suffer from heart or kidney failure are usually asked to reduce their fluid intake. If you are at all concerned, talk to your primary care doctor or a certified nutritionist about your particular needs. Most people get about eighty percent of their water from direct consumption; however, twenty percent of a person's water intake is consumed through the foods they eat. Foods that have a high water content include lettuce, watermelon, broccoli, and grapefruit. Each one of these foods is over ninety percent water. Carrots and apples also have a high water content. Drinking plain water is simply the best way to ensure that you are consuming your recommended daily supply of water, though. Filtered water from the tap is convenient and cost effective. If you want to add some flavor, you can add a squeeze of lime or lemon for a low-calorie cost-effective thirst quencher or try some exotic and affordable fruit infused water concoctions. Water is medicine and its use is important for the treatment or prevention of many diseases known to man.

8

T= Time with Family and Friends: Building Strong Relationships Could Prolong Your Life by 10 Years

So far, I have discussed with you many ways to live healthy lifestyles and covered a variety of physical aspects of health such as getting sufficient exercise, drinking plenty of water and eating a healthy, plant-based diet. However, health is a multi-faceted plane which involves not only our physical well-being but also our mental, emotional and spiritual well-being. A huge part of our health is the time we spend with our family, friends and strengthening our faith. Social relations are a complex subject and can mean many different things to many people. These bonds that we form and share become a part of who we are as individuals and are intrinsic to the type of quality of life that we experience as we get older. Research has proven that social ties are a fundamental part of a person's health. Relationships that are formed within the family unit are of utmost importance. In the Bible, we learned how God intended the family unit to function and how children should be raised. We are now seeing through evidence-based research how accurate these teachings truly are. Our friendships and those with whom we choose to associate ourselves are also important relationships. They help us to advance in life with peer-to-peer acceptance, knowledge, education and exercising our morals and values and growing as individuals as a result. In order to obtain good health, we cannot neglect the importance of the time that we need to spend with our family and good friends. In a few short minutes, we are going to go over some of the inner mechanics of how time with family and friends works within the overall health and healing process. But first, let's take a look at a broader example of how these structures relate to one another and to us as unique creations.

The Human Difference

Society, relationships, and even family are important aspects of nearly every creature's development. From dolphins and apes to the mighty lion and the noble wolf, we see how the interaction within the pride, pack or family gives everyone in the unit advantages that help it to thrive throughout its life. These relationships help to teach the younger generations survival skills and techniques, how to find mates and reproduce and helps to give them a sense of belonging and purpose within the unit. Even in the animal kingdom, we can see how social ties and bonds increase the survivability of these creatures.

In the Bible, it says that humans are created in the image of God; however, God is described as being so magnificent and fantastic that it is probable that physical characteristics are perhaps one of the least likely commonalities that humans have with their Creator. However, there are so many other characteristics that humans possess that distinctly set them apart from all of God's other creations. Anthropology is defined as the study of humankind, in particular. It is the comparative study of human societies, cultures, and their development. If one were to take a look at human societies of the distant past, we can clearly see how things such as creativity, consciousness, and even abstract thinking distinguish us from all other species on earth. As with these unique characteristics, our social relationships are also clearly different from animal species.

Social Relationships and Survivability

For centuries, humans have been studying the bonds and relationships that we form throughout our lives and how they impact us on a psychological and physiological level. In fact, research has proven that there is a direct connection between the impact that externally provided social support has on a person's longevity and their health outcomes. These studies conducted are designed to evaluate the benefits associated with how social connectedness correlates with happiness and it has been determined through this research that strong social bonds are associated with a fifty percent increased chance of survival over the course of the investigation on average.[1] To

107

put it into perspective, these tests reveal that a happy individual in an economically developed nation might live four to ten years longer than a person who is unhappy. Belonging to social groups and networks is actually reported to be just as important a predictor of health as are diet and exercise.[2] Regardless of what age group a person may belong to, social isolation is a dangerous and harmful situation. Particularly among seniors, social isolation is a known contributor in the development of chronic illnesses and has even been found to be as strong a factor in early death as smoking 15 cigarettes a day.[3] Communities that are age-friendly provide multitudinous opportunities for older adults to continue to contribute through certain types of civic engagement such as volunteering, being active in the political processes and even provide for suitable jobs.

Belonging and Purpose

Although there has been a lot of theory on the psychological and physiological processes of social integration and health outcomes for humans, critical evidence on the subject has only come about within the last ten to fifteen years according to psychology professor Bert Uchino at the University of Utah.[4] As a result, there is limited data to go by to give us a better understanding of the subject. Although researchers in the field are still unsure of exactly how social integration and relationships influence long life, there is no question that they are an integral part of a healthy outcome.

In a community where social connectedness is practiced, the inhabitants exhibit an increase in motivation, they display strong attributes of self-actualization, their self-esteem is enhanced and the children and youth gain a sense of belonging and purpose. During hard times or in tough situations, there is also a support network that is available to facilitate the healing and overcoming processes. The level of social connectedness that a person has access to throughout their life is a strong predictor of the quality of life that they may have. Some researchers even believe that it is a stronger predictor than the income or educational levels because personal happiness is more closely tied to these social bonds than income or education is.

Social contact is of fundamental importance to people because humans are social creatures. Isolation and loneliness have been known to contribute to poor outcomes in many health areas such as stress, anxiety or depression. Social isolation is also considered a risk factor for multiple chronic diseases, including obesity, high blood pressure, cancer, and diabetes.[5] Another important matter to note is that these increased health risks open the door for high-risk behaviors such as tobacco and alcohol use or a drastic reduction in healthy behaviors like eating well, exercising or getting adequate rest.

Happiness

The ancient Greeks came up with two approaches to what happiness is. The first is that happiness is a feeling of pleasure and is an emotion. The second is that happiness is about values such as kindness, generosity, and honesty and was less of an emotion and more of an idea. Today, modern scientists and theorists in the psychology of this phenomenon are finding that happiness is a mixture of both of these combined. One such theory suggests that there are six domains of human growth important to a person's overall well-being. The first domain is self-acceptance. The second is "the establishment of quality ties to others."[6] Social connection has been associated with feelings of positivity, and rejection and loneliness are perceived as negative according to Shelly Taylor at the University of California in Los Angeles. She suggests that stress due to relationship conflicts leads to increased inflammation levels in the body and can lead to more serious health issues.

Generosity is another social connection that research has shown to better one's physical and mental health. Research has linked different forms of generosity to increased health benefits in people with chronic illness, including HIV and multiple sclerosis and even among the elderly. In fact, professor of preventative medicine at Stony Brook University, Stephen Post, even included these results in his book "Why Good Things Happen to Good People."[7] Generosity has also been known to increase positive overall outlooks in people. When we are generous and give to others, there is a closeness that is experienced by both parties. Sonja Lyubomirsky, the author of "The How of Happiness," explains how acts of kindness lead us to perceive others more positively. Consequently, feelings of gratitude have been found to be integral to happiness, health, and social bonds.

The Impact of Early Social Connections

As research and technology advance, we are seeing increasing evidence that social connectedness is more of a determining factor than previously anticipated for both successes in life and even our mental health. For example, we have learned from neuroscience research that thought, emotions, and action occur through the activation of neural circuits in the brain. Through genetic makeup and learned experience, we are finding links to the wiring of these circuits. Children learn certain behaviors through their parents from young ages through the senses as well as genetic attributes that also contribute to their behavior and the circuitry connections within their brains.[8] Experts in social psychology recommend that active social connectedness begins as early as adolescence because this is when children are the most receptive, although there is a wide range of behaviors that can be learned as young as infancy.

It is a known fact that supportive and caring relationships within the family unit promote academic achievement in children all the way up through young adulthood. These connections also protect against involvement in health-risk behaviors by adolescents. The same holds true for in-school relationships with mentors such as teachers and school counselors who facilitate the learning process. Genuine support and care from school mentors promote higher levels of academic motivation and reduce the likelihood of the child participating in health-risk behaviors. School connectedness is a much broader conceptualization that requires much more extensive study because it involves more complicated relationships that are slightly less robust than family ties yet can cause long-term damage nonetheless. The construct combines perceptions of safety, support, trust, and belonging on a peer-to-peer basis whereas family connectedness involves parent-child and sibling-to-sibling relationships. This is generally the second level of social exposure that a child will encounter and has a tremendous impact on their development.

Studies show that positive school connectedness is associated with constructive mental health development and lower rates of involvement in multiple health-risk behaviors including substance use, sexual intercourse, violence, delinquency, and suicidality. The bonds that the students form in this stage of the development process and the peers that they choose to associate themselves with are usually based off of the foundation that is learned and experienced in the home. In any event, a searching young adult who has access to multiple social ties also has access to a variety of sources of information and thereby increases the likelihood of having access to an appropriate course of action to help foster relevant health behaviors or to minimize stressful or risky situations.

The Impact of Social Connections Later in Life

As I have talked about adolescent health and younger health affected by social connectedness, now I will focus on how social connectedness impacts elderly people's health and habits. All too often, we see elderly people who have fewer social contacts and oftentimes feel lonely. Many may feel forgotten or abandoned and as a result, their health, both psychological and physiological, also suffers. A study conducted by researchers shows that different types of leisure activities that elderly adults choose to participate in explain a significant part what their social connectedness level is and acts as a successful predictor of their physical state. If they are involved and engaged in activities such as voluntary work, cultural activities, holidays, sports, reading books, hobbies, and shopping, they are more likely to have a healthier outcome than those who do not get involved or engage themselves in productive and social activities. Local communities can develop age-friendly tactics and special programs to increase social connectedness and hence improve the quality of life for older adults. Having strong social connectedness within a community can lead to a more positive outcome for all the citizens residing within it, such as leisure participation and higher quality of life. Having positive social ties stimulates an individual to do certain activities because it facilitates social support.

Social Connections & Our Health

Earlier I briefly touched on some of the various health outcomes that can result from social connections and ties or a lack thereof. The scale is far and wide when it comes to how social interaction or isolation can influence a person. The key is in understanding the underlying mechanisms that are involved. A huge part of the issue is knowing that feelings of isolation and loneliness are like a double-edged sword. There are physical, emotional and mental complications all rolled into one multi-faceted problem and further research is showing us, now more than ever, how evident it is that we, as humans, all depend on each other in one way or another. For an average individual, social connectedness has been strongly associated with lower levels of blood pressure rates, better immune responses, and lower levels of stress hormones in the body. Each one of these qualities contributes to the prevention of chronic diseases and reinforces mental health.

Furthermore, there is considerable evidence to indicate that social connectedness can be especially helpful during times of significant stress. In fact, social interactions are themselves a potential uplift and a source of pleasure for most individuals. Within a family and/or community's connectedness lie core principles that allow successful recoveries from traumatic loss when catastrophic events occur. In contrast, one study showed that lack of social connection is a greater detriment to health than obesity, smoking, and high blood pressure.[9] There is also strong evidence to support the fact that those individuals who have social ties with others are able to more adequately over-come high-risk behaviors such as drug and/or alcohol addiction, smoking or poor eating habits. Addicts who have stronger support systems in place have a higher chance of kicking the habits than those who have no support at all.

Another important aspect of social connectedness that cannot be overlooked is the fact that researchers have discovered links between improved brain function and a delay in memory loss and social interaction. Lisa F. Berkman, director of the Harvard Center for Population and Development Studies, and her team of researchers found evidence to suggest that strong social ties, through friends, family and community groups, can preserve our brain health as we age and that social isolation may be an important risk factor for cognitive decline in the elderly. The finding appears in the July issue of *The American Journal of Public Health*. We know that social isolation increases a person's chances of being diagnosed with cognitive degenerative diseases such as Alzheimer's and dementia. On the other hand, social connectedness can increase brain activity and keep a person sharp for extended periods of time.

In Summary

As humans we were never meant to be alone, we need companionship. When this earth was created the Creator first created Adam, but then the idea for Adam to be left alone was not good, so Eve was created later. You see, we all need someone to socialize with. True health is not merely the absence of physical ailments but social and mental well-being is also important. Studies have shown that regular interactions with family and friends are vital for optimal health. Loneliness and social isolation or even weak social bonds are detrimental to your health. In fact, researchers believe that people with strong social support live 10 years longer than people who live alone without friends and family bonding.

Companionship and social bonds are such an intrinsic part of who we are that without them, other aspects of our lives also suffer such as our health, our mental capabilities, and our emotional state. In order to achieve total health and wellness we need to address all the aspects of healing besides just physical issues. The time we spend with our family and friends will not only prepare us for our journey throughout our lives, but also help us to cope with obstacles and setbacks along the way. Life was never intended to be easy, but with a little bit of faith along with the help and guidance from the relationships that we are blessed with, we are able to overcome and grow as strong and healthy individuals.

9

H= Happiness and Hope: A Merry Heart is Medicine

Could a positive thought process and a sunny outlook mean healthier communities? Could hope actually help fight heart disease and chronic migraines? Could being happy protect against illnesses like hypertension and diabetes? Is it true that happy people tend to live longer than those who are not – and if so, why? These are the kinds of questions that researchers are beginning to ask as they explore a new and sometimes unorthodox method of improving public health. Through thorough investigations and research, scientists and doctors are starting to document and understand the link between positive emotions and good health.

Certain physical responses, such as blood pressure, are considered to be involuntary, right? Although this is largely true, we do have a degree of conscious control over them as well. Many people, when they think of the concept of good health, forget that mental, emotional and spiritual well-being are a cornerstone of that concept. So many times we tend to get so caught up in daily life that we lose sight of the fact that our minds, emotions and spiritual connection to the Divine play a critical role in our health. Throughout our history, many healing systems have taken to the practice of interconnecting the mind, body, and spirit for whole-person healing. This includes Hippocrates, who is considered the father of modern medicine. He believed that good health was a balance of the mind, body, and even one's environment. Today the World **Health** Organization (WHO) **defined Health** as being "a state of complete physical, mental, and social well-being and not merely the absence of disease or infirmity."

There are scores of scientific breakthroughs that have illuminated the mind-body connection in health. These breakthroughs have directly translated into effective therapies that support a patient's journey through healthier lifestyles and longevity. We have even observed how virtually every major medical center now has some sort of mind-body program, such as support groups, woven into their patients' medical treatment. This is especially common with serious illnesses such as heart disease and cancer.

Stress is a Killer

Many medical conditions that are a result of our mind-body connection are oftentimes related to other diseases and symptoms. One of the biggest and most widely known culprits is stress. In 1936, a Hungarian-born doctor by the name of Hans Selye began researching the issues of stress and how it affects a person's health. Through his research and study at the Université de Montréal, he was able to describe how the long-term effects of constant stress could affect us on a biological and physiological level. Because of his efforts and his numerous contributions to the field, we now have a better understanding of how stress can adversely affect our health.[1] According to Harvard Medical School and Harvard Health Publications, some scientists are even investigating whether prolonged stress factors can actually take a toll on the immune system itself and decrease our ability to fight disease.[2] Dr. Robert Ader, Ph.D., who was a professor emeritus of Psychiatry at the University of Rochester Medical Center and founder of the new field of psychoneuroimmunology, provided a link between the brain, behavior, and immune function. His theory was that the human mind could actually increase immune function and assist with the prevention and reversal of illness.[3] Likewise, the mind could also decrease immune function and leave people susceptible to chronic conditions – many of which are life-threatening. Such conditions could include:

- Migraines
- Heart disease
- Obesity
- Diabetes
- Depression and anxiety
- Gastrointestinal problems
- Irritable bowel syndrome (IBS)
- Accelerated aging
- Premature death

119

These conditions can be a direct result of the wear-and-tear of stress on a person's life. This is only a brief overview but the list goes on and on.[4] A person's thought process could be the difference between health and disease. Thirty years ago, Dr. Ader's theories were met with skepticism, but today, they are studied and applied by researchers in a wide array of medical specialties around the world.

Healing Vs. Curing

Stress tends to have an adverse effect on your health and overall wellbeing. When a person is under stress, it can be difficult to "look on the bright side." Sometimes, circumstances may seem grim and dreary. But negative emotions are only half of the equation. Fortunately for us, there are things that can be done to help us to do just that – to look on the bright side of things and think positively. Actively taking part in de-stressing activities can help to balance out the pressures of daily life, such as work, chores, responsibilities and other challenges. Exercise, prayer, and meditation are a few things that have been proven to reduce a person's stress levels and help them to achieve better health outcomes. In fact, scientists and researchers are beginning to realize through various tests in numerous fields, that positive thinking is about much more than just having an optimistic attitude. Thoughts that focus on positivity can actually create real value in a person's life. Barbara Fredrickson is a positive psychology researcher at the University of North Carolina, and her work is among the most referenced and cited in her field. She talks about how being positive, and choosing to be happy and to have hope can actually provide whole body "healing" to a person and not just a "cure."

The way we think and our thought processes can actually determine, in part, our health outcomes. This is proven by the placebo effect where a pseudo treatment is used in place of actual treatment such as a sugar pill being administered in place of an actual prescription drug. Findings reveal that an average of 44% of subjects tested through this method has shown positive responses. The cause of these responses is not necessarily physical but mental and these results strengthen the position of the mind-body connection and how a cheerful outlook can help us to overcome certain health challenges.

To further drive this point home, let me give you a real-life example. Associate professor of psychiatry and medicine at the University of Pittsburgh's Cancer Institute, Dr. Sandra Levy, discovered that women with a hopeful and positive outlook had an increased chance of survival as opposed to those women who had lost hope or become discouraged.[5] Some scientists speculate that the root cause of this is because of the fact that when we experience negative emotions such as anger, fear, frustration and stress, they send signals to the brain which in turn stimulates the endocrine system to release hormones that have an adverse effect on the immune cell's ability to divide. This results in a decline in immune function which can lead to an increased risk of becoming susceptible to illness. This process is very similar to what happens in the "Fight-or-Flight" process.

Prayer and Meditation

Now that we have a greater understanding of how the mind-body connection works, how can we retrain our minds and thought processes to think more positively and focus on things such as being happy and hopeful? While Dr. Selye was investigating how stress affected the human body, Harvard cardiologist Dr. Herbert Benson, MD, was studying the other side of the spectrum which he called the "relaxation response." Dr. Benson demonstrated that, by doing relaxing activities such as prayer and meditation, we can bring about physiological changes in our bodies including a lower heart rate, lower breathing rate, and decreased muscle tension along with positive changes in brain waves.[6]

Breakthroughs in our understanding of the mind-body connection have translated into effective therapies for treating these many stress-related disorders as well as supporting a patient's journey through illnesses and trauma. Having hope and happiness in our lives is a powerful way to maintain a positive outlook and successfully weather the trials which come to all of us in life. It helps us on a spiritual, emotional and mental level as well as a physiological one too. The relationship between prayer and health has been the subject of scores of studies over the past forty years. Dr. Andrew Newberg, director of the Center for Spirituality and the Mind at the University of Pennsylvania, also found that prayer and meditation increase levels of dopamine, which is associated with states of well-being and joy.[7]

Although it may not seem like you are making a big difference in your health, or even if you "think" that you could be doing something "better" with your time, you need to take some time out to focus on mental, emotional and spiritual healing. Going to church or sitting silently and praying or meditating can do wonders for our physical health and spiritual well-being and we need to make sure that we make time for these important activities. As time passes, we will slowly begin to retrain our mind to a more positive thought process and it will become second nature.

In Summary

Another important aspect of living lives filled with happiness and hope is that we need to remember to surround ourselves with positive people who can help us along our journey, encourage us and believe with us when we are faced with obstacles. The Bible says, "And let us not neglect our meeting together, as some people do, but encourage one another." Two thousand years ago, people understood the importance of a strong and resilient support group. As we move towards a lifestyle of health, happiness, and hope, we need to make sure that we bring others with us and have other like-minded individuals supporting us as well. Our spiritual health is an integral part of being wholly healthy. That begins by working on and taking time for our spiritual selves. As a physician, my goal for all of my patients is whole-person health, not just physical health — healing and not just curing. It is one thing to cure some symptoms, but it is a completely different thing to heal the whole person from the inside out. Having a spiritual connection to the Divine can greatly increase a person's positive outlook on life and offer the kind of healthy lifestyle that *true* happiness and hope can bring.

10

Y= Yield Years of Abundant Life

Aging and death are inevitable processes of life, yet there are those who fear these natural processes. Aging has long been associated with pain, illness, and frailty. However, there are those who are turning the tables on the aging process and early death and living longer, healthier and more abundant lives. I have already discussed with you a few of them through this journey together. People like Diana Nyad and Ernistine Shepard are changing what it means to be a senior citizen, but they are not the only ones. There are average, everyday people just like you and me, who are not in the Guinness Book of World Records or in the news, yet they are living long and abundant lives even past one hundred years old. There is a higher incidence of people living beyond 100 years in some specific regions in the world such as Sardinia (Italy), Loma Linda (California), Nicoya (Costa Rica), Okinawa (Japan), and Icaria (Greece). These people (centenarians, as they are often referred to) are living proof that living longer and healthier is attainable if you follow certain guidelines, most of which were mentioned in the previous chapters of this book.

If you are a person of faith then you will agree that many years ago when this world was first created life was simple then, people's diet was different and the lifespan was way above that of today. The Bible reports that the longest liver enjoyed more than 900 years of life; however, there is still hope today to live way beyond 100 years if you adhere to the principles that I have laid out in this book. Through interviews conducted with many of these centenarians, it has been discovered that most of them have one thing in common – similar habits. They share the same type of diet with a high abundance of fruits, vegetables, nuts, seeds and whole grains, they live a very active lifestyle, and they enjoy a stress-free lifestyle and have faith. Today there is a wealth of research to confirm that the practice of healthy lifestyle habits will indeed propel the prevention and reversal of chronic diseases.

The Most Important Step

In general, we all practice habits which will ultimately lead to poor health and early death. Even though the consequences of our choices are obvious, you would agree with me that habits are usually hard to break away from. However, as you consider this journey one of the most important steps that you will have to take is understanding why you need to make the change, and defining your strategies to success. In chapter one, I showed how "impossibilities" became possible. Now if you were ever told in the past that your disease process is irreversible or if you think you can never get off your medications, know that there is hope. Many people have used these same principles and are now enjoying better health. I indeed have some of those same people in my practice. Many health-care providers are now recommending these same principles to their patients; however, some people find it very difficult to follow through.

Doctors such as T. Colin Campbell, John McDougall, and others have been using some of these same principles with their patients for many years. I urge you to assess your current overall health then take action. Taking the first step is oftentimes the hardest, but the rewards far outweigh the difficulties. The centenarians of our generation are examples of what taking that first step can do for all the rest of us hoping to achieve longevity. Don't put good habits, especially healthy eating habits, off any longer. When it comes to formulating good habits, we have to remember that the most important step is the first one.

Setting Up for Success

Here success means reversing your chronic medical condition. It means losing weight, keeping that weight off and finally having that high self-esteem that you longed for. To some, success might be just getting off all those pills that you were told that you would be on for the rest of your life, or just having the ability to live your life without the fear of dying early. All these goals are possible. Let's recap on some of the information mentioned in the earlier chapters of this book. Many studies have confirmed that simple measures such as spending time in nature are essential in disease prevention and reversal. Adequate exposure to sunlight will:

1. Decrease blood pressure.
2. Treat depression.
3. Improve mental alertness.
4. Improve bone health and decrease the risk of osteoporosis.
5. Decrease your risk of dying young.

You see, it is not difficult to succeed in attaining long-lasting health and wellness. You may just need to make few subtle changes in your lifestyle. Let's focus on something as simple as rest. Imagine yourself working twenty-four hours daily for one month without taking time to rest. What impact would that have on your health or would that even be possible, no sleep for a month? Studies show that the longest a person could possibly survive without sleep is about three days. You can now agree that adequate rest will produce health and prevent early death. Now there are two rest cycles: daily rest and weekly rest. Everyone needs at least 7-9 hours of daily rest as well as weekly rest. You must take off one day weekly to restore, reset, replenish and rejuvenate the mind, body, and the spirit. Here are the some of the health successes of adequate rest.

1. Build stronger immune system.
2. Restoration and reparation of the cells and tissues of the body.
3. Decrease high blood pressure and the risk of heart disease.
4. Decrease the risk of obesity.
5. Improve mood.
6. Improve memory.
7. Decrease the risk of Alzheimer's.
8. Improve one's mental alertness and focus.
9. Add years to your life.

As we continue to recap on the gains that you will obtain from following the principles that I have given in the previous chapters, let us turn our focus on the appetite. There is no secret now. Everyone is well aware that what you put in your mouth will either prolong or shorten your life. The great father of medicine, Hippocrates, said, "Let food be thy medicine and thy medicine be food." This is powerful but indeed true. The wise Thomas Edison echoed a similar sentiment many years ago. "The doctor of the future will give no medication, but will interest his patients in the care of the human frame, diet and in the cause and prevention of disease."

Fit for Life

Obtaining regular physical exercise has now been prescribed by healthcare providers. It has become the next habit to practice for all those that desire to be free of all diseases including cancer. Adequate exercise is also a crucial aspect of a healthy lifestyle. Paired with good nutrition, you have a recipe for success and longevity. The centenarians that we discussed earlier all practice some form of regular physical activity, even if it is just gardening, walking in nature or swimming. The goal is not to be the strongest or the fastest – the goal is to be healthy.

Some habits that are contrary to being healthy are sitting on the sofa and watching television when you get home. Although it may seem tempting to plop down on the couch after a long and grueling day at work and flip on your favorite T.V. show, going for a leisurely walk with the dog or taking the bike out on a trail will actually give you more energy than "resting" in front of the television. Our nation is currently experiencing an epidemic of chronic illnesses that consist of diseases such as diabetes, heart disease, and obesity. Even our children are being diagnosed with these illnesses that, in the past, were considered to be adult conditions. The statistics that we are faced with today are staggering. In fact, if these trends continue, experts believe that one (1) in every three (3) people will develop diabetes in their lifetime – that is one-third of the world's population.

If we want to change the destructive path that we are on, it has to begin with us and the way we choose to live our lives. By spending at least thirty minutes every day doing some form of exercise or physical activity, we can bring down these numbers considerably. When we think of the big picture and our health, thirty minutes a day spent on physical activity is not all that impossible a sacrifice to make, especially if we are doing something that we actually enjoy. No one ever said that physical activity and exercise had to be work. If that were the case, I highly doubt that anyone would do it at all. We can make exercise a fun experience by being creative. Go for walks with your friends or a bike ride with your kids, take a swimming class or pick up gardening as a hobby. You could even grow your own organic food in your own garden. That guarantees that your food is always fresh and free of commercial pesticides and other potentially harmful chemicals. The best part about gardening is that you do not need a lot of space or land. You can grow small crops such as herbs, potatoes, and tomatoes easily on a balcony, porch or kitchen counter. Before beginning any type of physical exercise regimen, it is important to consult with your primary care physician first. So here are some health benefits that regular physical exercise will yield:

1. Cure diabetes.
2. Cure obesity.
3. Build stronger bones.
4. Improve blood pressure.
5. Improve Mood.
6. Decrease cholesterol.
7. Build endurance.
8. Reduce the risk of some cancers.
9. Decrease disability.
10. Add years to your life.

Keep Your Health in Check

The notion of completely handing your health to your doctor for success and longevity is not the smart way to go. Each person must be empowered to ensure good healthcare outcomes. Partnership with a healthcare provider is important and valuable. You will need to have routine health screenings which are important for early detection of diseases. The goal standard is prevention; however, early detection of diseases is essential for adequate and better outcome. So here is the summary:

1. Annual Physical Evaluation: You should schedule regular visits with your healthcare provider, at least once per year. During this visit, you should discuss the need for vaccines as well as the need for preventive health screenings that are relevant for your age group.
2. Blood Pressure screening: This begins at age 20 years and continues at least yearly.
3. Cholesterol: (fasting lipid profile) This should begin as early as age 21 years.
4. Glucose: Fasting blood glucose evaluation should begin at 45 years but given the incidence of diabetes I suggest that this should be done earlier.
5. Mammogram: This study screens for breast cancer. All women at age 40 years should have the first mammogram and yearly thereafter.
6. PSA (prostate specific antigen) Digital rectal exam: These tests screen for prostate cancer. Men should

begin to be screened for prostate cancer at age 40 years.

7. Colon cancer screening: This test should begin at age 50 years in those people without a family history of colon cancer. However, if there is a history of colon cancer in the family then the screening should begin 10 years earlier than the age the youngest person in the family was diagnosed with the cancer. (For example, if the mother was diagnosed at age 40 years with colon cancer, then everyone should begin to be screened at age 30 years.)

8. Pap smear screens for cancer of the cervix in women: This test should begin at about age 21 if the woman is sexually active and continue every 3 years thereafter. The test is not done after age 65-70 years, or in patients who have had hysterectomies.

Statistics show that early detection of disease will reduce the incidence of death. For example, early detection of breast cancer may decrease the risk of dying from the disease by 25-30%.

Having adequate access to healthcare can increase a person's ability to live a long and healthy life and even their quality of life. It is equally important to report any changes or medical concerns that you are experiencing to your primary care physician as soon as you notice them. These changes could be the first signs of a potential health risk.

A Purpose-Driven Life

Let's stop for a few minutes and take some time to practice a simple exercise together. You don't need to over-analyze this exercise, but you do need, to be honest with yourself in order for it to work. With this exercise, we are going to evaluate the impact that our mental or spiritual well-being has on our physical and emotional health and how living a life of purpose can drive us as human beings. I want you to think about one of your happiest moments in life thus far. It needs to be a moment when you felt truly connected, when you were exactly where you needed to be, doing exactly what you were born to do in that instant. Remember how that felt? Remember the warmth inside, almost like a soft glow? What were you doing? Who were you with? The answers to these questions are extremely important in finding purpose in our lives.

Hopefully, most of you who tried this exercise can actually think back upon a moment like this and smile at the memory. Obtaining and maintaining wholesome health encompasses a healthy body, mind, and spirit. In this journey to attain health, happiness, longevity and abundant life all aspects of health must be addressed. Many studies have shown that social connectedness is essential. People who have good social support, strong family bonds, and good friends tend to enjoy better health. However, those who lack social support die an average of 10 years younger. Scientists have also discovered that people who are optimistic, those who see the glass half full, those who are happy and hopeful tend to be healthier and live longer. People of faith who belong to a faith community tend to have less incidence of depression, anxiety, suicide and chronic illness.

My Desire for You

So having read the pages of this book have you found what you are searching for? What is your purpose in life? Is it attaining physical health, emotional health or could it be a spiritual connection? I know what I would like you to have and that is for you to enjoy your fullest potential! Physical health is only a part of my desire for you. In John 10:10 it reads, "The thief comes not but for to kill, steal and destroy but I come that they might have life and have it more abundantly," and in 3 John 2: it reads, "Beloved, I wish above all things that thou mayest prosper and be in health, even as thy soul prospereth."

It is my desire that as you follow these basic pillars of health you will find complete health, wholeness, peace, happiness, hope and abundant life. The Creator wants you to prosper in health, both for the body and soul. This also is my wish for you. Please empower those whom you meet on your journey to amazing health and longevity.

Acknowledgements

I would like to extend my sincerest thanks and gratitude to Christina E. Phillips for the longs hours spent in researching some of the material needed to make this book a reality.

How could I even begin to thank Pastor Randrick Chance and the team at Strategic Secrets for the many hours of coaching and encouragement on getting this book completed? Thank you very much. May God always richly bless your ministry.

Many thanks also to my staff and patients. You are the reason we get up every day to do what we do. Thanks for allowing me to serve you and thanks for supporting our mission and vision.

I especially thank you for reading this book and for the success I know you will have when you practice these secret pillars daily. Don't give up on your health goals. Improve your lifestyle habits, even in small increments and you will be blessed with health for the rest of your life. Thanks for sharing this journey with me. I pray and wish you all the best. If there's anything else I can do to help you, head over to www.Gethealthywithdrcooper.tv, www.Cooperinternalmedicine.com, or visit us at one of our locations mentioned on the back cover of this book.

About the Author

Dona Cooper-Dockery, M.D., is a physician, author, and speaker who has dedicated over 25 years to positively changing healthcare outcomes both nationally and internationally. She is board-certified in internal medicine and holds active memberships in the American Academy of Lifestyle Medicine and the American Medical Association. She wrote the health study series, *My Health and The Creator*, and also writes for and produces the health magazine, *Get Healthy*. Her latest book, *Fourteen Days to Amazing Health*, outlines various success strategies that will empower readers to take control of their health, believe that there is an alternative to medications, change their paradigm, and a live happier, healthier, and more fulfilled life.

Dr. Cooper-Dockery is also the founder and director of *Cooper Internal Medicine and* the *Cooper Wellness and Disease Prevention Center* where patients are not only diagnosed and treated using traditional healthcare approaches, but she also emphasizes uprooting the causes of chronic diseases through lifestyle modifications. Her highly effective 12 weeks to wellness program has had significant life-changing results on her patients. Many of whom are enjoying more health with less medication, some have even gotten off medication entirely! These patients have reversed diabetes, improved blood pressure, others have lost weight, reduced cholesterol, or decrease the risk of coronary artery disease and early death.

She is actively engaged in various communities providing healthy lifestyle seminars and free medical care, not only in the USA but also in countries such as Haiti, Jamaica, the Philippines, and Europe. She is the host of the popular TV show, *Get Healthy with Dr. Cooper*, which airs bi-weekly on two local TV channels. To learn more about Dr. Cooper-Dockery or to get health resources, please visit www.Cooperinternalmedicine.com and www.Gethealthywithdrcooper.tv.

Resources

For more information, tools, and resources to help you get healthy for life, go to www.Gethealthywithdrcooper.com/resources.

For her growing library of videos, literature, courses, and community initiatives, visit www.Gethealthywithdrcooper.tv. There, you can also get Dr. Cooper-Dockery's latest book, *Fourteen Days to Amazing Health* and her study guides, *My Health and The Creator*.

For personalized coaching, questions, or advice, contact her private practice at www.Cooperinternatmedicine.com or visit one of the locations mentioned on the back cover.

Endnotes

Chapter One References:

[1] Sparacino, A. (n.d.). Top 10 Healthiest New Year's Resolutions - Health.com. Retrieved from http://www.health.com/health/gallery/0,,20452233,00.html

[2] Kirkham, E. (2015, December 31). "Enjoying Life to the Fullest" Is 2016's Top Resolution | TIME. Retrieved from http://time.com/money/4163867/top-new-years-resolution-2016/

[3] Hill, N. (1999). Think and grow rich: Teaching, for the first time, the famous Andrew Carnegie formula for money-making, based upon the thirteen proven steps to riches. Retrieved from http://eventualmillionaire.com/Resources/ThinkandGrowRich.pdf

*[4] NutritionED.org. (n.d.). The Vegan and Vegetarian Approaches to Nutrition and Dietetics. Retrieved from http://www.nutritioned.org/vegan-vegetarian-approaches.html

[5] Mergenthaler, P., Lindauer, U., Dienel, G. A., & Meisel, A. (2013). Sugar for the brain: the role of glucose in physiological and pathological brain function. Trends in Neurosciences, 36(10), 587–597. http://doi.org/10.1016/j.tins.2013.07.001

[6] Diabetes UK. (2009, October 2). Diabetes and obesity rates soar - Diabetes UK. Retrieved from

https://www.diabetes.org.uk/About_us/
News_Landing_Page/Diabetes-and-obesity-rates-soar/
[7] Centers for Disease Control and Prevention. (2014, October 24). 2014 Statistics Report | Data & Statistics | Diabetes | CDC. Retrieved from http://www.cdc.gov/diabetes/data/statistics/2014statisticsreport.html
[8] American Diabetes Association. (n.d.). Statistics About Diabetes: American Diabetes Association®. Retrieved from http://www.diabetes.org/diabetes-basics/statistics/

Chapter Two References:

[2] Earth Policy Institute. (2012, August). Eco-Economy Indicators - Forest Cover | EPI. Retrieved from http://www.earth-policy.org/indicators/C56
[4] Strong's Concordance. (n.d.). Strong's Hebrew Lexicon Search Results. Retrieved from http://www.eliyah.com/cgi-bin/strongs.cgi?file=hebrewlexicon&isindex=2896
[5] Reinberg, S. (2016, January). Sunlight Might Be Good for Your Blood Pressure: Study — WebMD. Retrieved from http://www.webmd.com/hypertension-high-blood-pressure/news/20140120/sunlight-might-be-good-for-your-blood-pressure-study
[6] Nall, R., LaFlamme, M., & Healthline. (2015, November 9). What Are the Benefits of Sunlight? Retrieved from http://www.healthline.com/health/depression/benefits-sunlight
[7] Medical News Today. (2004, August 25). Cigarette smoke produces 10 times more air pollution than diesel car exhaust

- Medical News Today. Retrieved from
http://www.medicalnewstoday.com/releases/12481.php

[8] Enviro-Lite Solutions. (2016). Enviro-Lite Solutions,
LLC. Retrieved from http://www.enviro-litesolutions.
com/#!people/e623h

[9] Faris, S., & Krucik, M.D., G. (2014, August 12). Is Depression
Genetic or Environmental? Retrieved from
http://www.healthline.com/health/depression/
genetic#Overview1

[10] Perina, K. (2003, January 1). Misery Loves Company
| Psychology Today. Retrieved from https://
www.psychologytoday.com/articles/200301/
misery-loves-company

[11] Griffin, M. (n.d.). Laughter: Good For Your Health - WebMD.
Retrieved from http://www.webmd.com/balance/features/
give-your-body-boost-with-laughter?page=2

Chapter Three References:

[1] Baumgartner Law Firm. (n.d.). Drowsy Driving – Common
Cause of Semi-Truck Accidents. Retrieved from
https://www.hg.org/article.asp?id=298sixsix

[2] The Farber Law Group. (n.d.). Bellevue, Washington Auto Crash
Lawyer: Drowsy Driving Accidents: Seattle, Washington Car
Accident Attorney. Retrieved from http://www.hgfarber.
com/drowsy-driving-accidents.html

[3] Federal Motor Carrier Safety Administration. (2014, April 9).
New Hours-of-Service Safety Regulations to Reduce Truck
Driver Fatigue Begin Today | Federal Motor Carrier Safety
Administration. Retrieved from https://www.fmcsa.dot.

gov/newsroom/new-hours-service-safety-regulations-reduce-truck-driver-fatigue-begin-today

[4] The Farber Law Group. (n.d.). Bellevue, Washington Auto Crash Lawyer: Drowsy Driving Accidents: Seattle, Washington Car Accident Attorney. Retrieved from http://www.hgfarber.com/drowsy-driving-accidents.html

[5] National Sleep Foundation. (n.d.). Improve Your Memory with a Good Night's Sleep. Retrieved from https://sleepfoundation.org/sleep-news/improve-your-memory-good-nights-sleep

[6] OECD. (201six, March 14). Average annual hours actually worked per worker. Retrieved from https://stats.oecd.org/Index.aspx?DataSetCode=ANHRS

[7] USA Today, & Hess, A. (2013, June 8). On holiday: Countries with the most vacation days. Retrieved from http://www.usatoday.com/story/money/business/2013/06/08/countries-most-vacation-days/2400193/

[8] Medical Research News. (2008, January 9). Stress causes whole body deterioration. Retrieved from http://www.news-medical.net/news/2008/01/09/34154.aspx

[9] Lam, M. (n.d.). Don't let Stage 3 Adrenal Fatigue ruin your life. Retrieved from https://www.drlam.com/articles/adrenalexhaustion.asp

[10] Robinson, J. (2015, March 1). The Symptoms of Addison's Disease. Retrieved from http://www.webmd.com/a-to-z-guides/understanding-addisons-disease-symptoms

[11] The National Institute of Diabetes and Digestive and Kidney Diseases. (n.d.). Overweight and Obesity Statistics. Retrieved from http://www.niddk.nih.gov/health-information/health-statistics/Pages/overweight-obesity-statistics.aspx

[12] National Sleep Foundation. (2015, February 2). National Sleep Foundation Recommends New Sleep Durations. Retrieved from https://sleepfoundation.org/media-center/press-release/national-sleep-foundation-recommends-new-sleep-times

[13] Robinson, J. (2014, October 22). Stages of Sleep: REM and Non-REM Sleep Cycles. Retrieved from http://www.webmd.com/sleep-disorders/guide/sleep-101

[14] Mayo Clinic. (2014, June 9). Sleep tips: 7 steps to better sleep - Mayo Clinic. Retrieved from http://www.mayoclinic.org/healthy-lifestyle/adult-health/in-depth/sleep/art-20048379

Chapter Four References:

[1] BBC. (n.d.). BBC - History - Historic Figures: James Lind (1716 - 1794). Retrieved from http://www.bbc.co.uk/history/historic_figures/lind_james.shtml

[2] Christiaan Eijkman, Beriberi and Vitamin B1. Nobelprize.org. Nobel Media AB 2014. Web. 22 Mar 2016. Retrieved from http://www.nobelprize.org/educational/medicine/vitamin_b1/eijkman.html

[3] Sir Frederick Gowland Hopkins. (2016). In Encyclopedia Britannica. Retrieved from http://www.britannica.com/biography/Frederick-Gowland-Hopkins

[4] Centers for Disease Control and Prevention. (2015, March 31). IMMPaCt: Micronutrient Facts | DNPAO | CDC. Retrieved from http://www.cdc.gov/immpact/micronutrients/

[5] Kim, S., & Radecki, J. (n.d.). Nutrients. Retrieved from http://www.diet.com/g/nutrients

[6] Harvard Health Publications. (n.d.). Vitamins & Minerals: Are You Getting What You Need? Retrieved from http://www. helpguide.org/harvard/vitamins-and-minerals.htm

[7] Butler, N. (2015, November 6). Nutritional Deficiencies (Malnutrition). Retrieved from http://www.healthline.com/ health/malnutrition

[8] Kim, S., & Radecki, J. (n.d.). Nutrients. Retrieved from http://www.diet.com/g/nutrients

[9] World Health Organization (n.d.). Micronutrient deficiencies. Retrieved from http://www.who.int/nutrition/topics/ida/ en/

Chapter Five References:

[1] Brandt, M. (2004, July 21). Obese parents increase kids' risk of being overweight. Retrieved from http://news.stanford.edu/ news/2004/july21/med-obesity-721.html

[2] Campaign to End Obesity. (n.d.). The Campaign to End Obesity. Retrieved from http://www.obesitycampaign.org/obesity_ facts.asp

[3] Spark. (n.d.). Studies Show that Physically Active Kids Perform Better Academically. Retrieved from http://www.sparkpe.org/blog/ study-physically-active-kids-perform-better-academically/

[4] American Diabetes Association. (n.d.). Diabetes Myths: American Diabetes Association®. Retrieved from www.diabetes.org/diabetes-basics/myths/?referrer= https://www.google.com/

[5] Boehlke, J. (2015, October 19). How Does Exercise Improve Work Productivity? | LIVESTRONG.COM. Retrieved from http://www.livestrong.com/article/422836-how-does-exercise-improve-work-productivity/

[6] MU News Bureau. (2011, August 23). MU News Bureau | MU News Bureau. Retrieved from http://munews.missouri.edu/news-releases/2011/0823-mu-study-links-inactivity-with-risk-factors-for-type-2-diabetes/

[7] American Cancer Society. (n.d.). Diet and Physical exercise: What's the Cancer Connection? Retrieved from http://www.cancer.org/cancer/cancercauses/dietandphysicalactivity/diet-and-physical-activity

[8] Hathaway, B. (2015, March 2). New fat cells created quickly, but losing them .... Retrieved from news.yale.edu/2015/03/02/new-fat-cells-created-quickly-losing-them

[9] US National Library of Medicine. (2009). Exercise improves fat metabolism in muscle but does not increase 24-h fat oxidation. Retrieved from http://www.ncbi.nlm.nih.gov/pmc/articles/PMC2885974/

[10] Office of Disease Prevention and Health Promotion. (n.d.). Physical exercise Guidelines - health.gov. Retrieved from http://health.gov/paguidelines/

[11] Harvard. (n.d.). Physical exercise guidelines: How much exercise do you need? – The Nutrition Source – Harvard T.H. Chan School of Public Health. Retrieved from http://www.hsph.harvard.edu/nutritionsource/2013/11/20/physical-activity-guidelines-how-much-exercise-do-you-need/

[12] Mayo Clinic. (n.d.). Exercise intensity: How to measure it - Mayo Clinic. Retrieved from http://www.mayoclinic.

org/healthy-lifestyle/fitness/in-depth/exercise-intensity/
art-20046887

[13] Health.gov. (n.d.). Chapter 1 - 2008 Physical exercise
Guidelines - health.gov. Retrieved from http://health.gov/
paguidelines/guidelines/chapter1.aspx

Chapter Six References:

[1] Cancer Research UK. (2015, April 2). Why is early diagnosis
important? | Cancer Research UK. Retrieved from
http://www.cancerresearchuk.org/about-cancer/
cancer-symptoms/why-is-early-diagnosis-important

[2] Alzheimer's & Dementia Alliance of Wisconsin. (n.d.).
Importance of an early diagnosis. Retrieved from
http://www.alzwisc.org/Importance%20of%20an%20
early%20diagnosis.htm

[3] American Diabetes Association. (2012). Statistics
About Diabetes: American Diabetes Association®.
Retrieved from www.diabetes.org/diabetes-basics/
statistics/?referrer=https://www.google.com/

[4] American Heart Association. (2014, December 19). High blood
pressure causing more deaths despite drop in heart disease,
stroke deaths - News on Heart.org. Retrieved from
http://news.heart.org/high-blood-pressure-causing-deaths-
despite-drop-heart-disease-stroke-deaths/

[5] The American Cancer Society. (n.d.). American Cancer Society
Guidelines for the Early Detection of Cancer. Retrieved
from http://www.cancer.org/healthy/findcancerearly/
cancerscreeningguidelines/american-cancer-society-
guidelines-for-the-early-detection-of-cancer

[6] The College of Physicians of Philadelphia. (2016, January 29). Different Types of Vaccines — History of Vaccines. Retrieved from http://www.historyofvaccines.org/content/articles/different-types-vaccines

[7] Office of Disease Prevention and Health Promotion. (n.d.). Access to Health Services | Healthy People 2020. Retrieved from https://www.healthypeople.gov/2020/topics-objectives/topic/Access-to-Health-Services

Chapter Seven References:

[1] USGS. (2016, May 2). How much water is there on Earth, from the USGS Water Science School. Retrieved from http://water.usgs.gov/edu/earthhowmuch.html

[2] Scientific American, & Lieberson, A. (2004, November 8). How long can a person survive without food? - Scientific American. Retrieved from http://www.scientificamerican.com/article/how-long-can-a-person-sur/

[3] Mayo Clinic. (2014, February). Dehydration Symptoms - Mayo Clinic. Retrieved from http://www.mayoclinic.org/diseases-conditions/dehydration/basics/symptoms/con-20030056

[4] Occupational Safety & Health Administration. (n.d.). Safety and Health Topics | Occupational Heat Exposure - Heat-related Illnesses and First Aid. Retrieved from https://www.osha.gov/SLTC/heatstress/heat_illnesses.html

[5] Centers for Disease Control and Prevention. (2011, June 20). CDC - Extreme Heat and Your Health: Warning Signs and

Symptoms of Heat Illness. Retrieved from http://www.cdc.gov/extremeheat/warning.html

[6] Burch, D. (2009, January 10). When Childbirth Was Natural, and Deadly. Retrieved from http://www.livescience.com/3210-childbirth-natural-deadly.html

[7] Healthline. (n.d.). Puerperal Infection | Definition & Patient Education. Retrieved from http://www.healthline.com/health/puerperal-infection#Overview1

[8] NPR Science Desk. (2015, January 12). The Doctor Who Championed Hand-Washing And Briefly Saved Lives: Shots - Health News: NPR. Retrieved from http://www.npr.org/sections/health-shots/2015/01/12/375663920/the-doctor-who-championed-hand-washing-and-saved-women-s-lives

[9] Natural Therapy Pages. (2008, September 20). Hydrotherapy - How it works & The Benefits of Hydrotherapy. Retrieved from http://www.naturaltherapypages.com.au/article/hydrotherapy

Chapter Eight References:

[1] Umberson, D., & Montez, J. K. (2010). Social Relationships and Health: A Flashpoint for Health Policy. Journal of Health and Social Behavior, 51(Suppl), S54–S66. http://doi.org/10.1177/0022146510383501

[2] Social Relationships and Health: A Flashpoint for Health Policy. (n.d.). Retrieved from http://www.ncbi.nlm.nih.gov/pmc/articles/PMC3150158/

[3] Miller, A. (2014, January). Friends wanted. Retrieved from http://www.apa.org/monitor/2014/01/cover-friends.aspx

[4] Blue, L. (2010, July 28). Wide Social Networks Are Key to Good Health, Says Study - TIME. Retrieved from http://content.time.com/time/health/article/0,8599,2006938,00.html

[5] Wilder Research. (2012, March). Social Connectedness and Health. Retrieved from https://www.bcbsmnfoundation.org/system/asset/resource/pdf_file/5/Social_Connectedness_and_Health.pd

[6] PsyBlog. (2014, April 3). The Key to Happiness: Brainpower or Social Connectedness? - PsyBlog. Retrieved from http://www.spring.org.uk/2014/04/the-key-to-happiness-brainpower-or-social-connectedness.php

[7] Marsh, J., & Suttie, J. (2010, December). 5 Ways Giving Is Good for You | Greater Good. Retrieved from http://greatergood.berkeley.edu/article/item/5_ways_giving_is_good_for_you

[8] REPSSI. (2014, May). Social Connectedness: The Power of Meaningful Relationships | REPSSI : Regional Psychosocial Support Initiative. Retrieved from http://www.repssi.org/social-connectedness-the-power-of-meaningful-relationships/

[9] Wilder Research. (2012, March). Social Connectedness and Health. Retrieved from https://www.bcbsmnfoundation.org/system/asset/resource/pdf_file/5/Social_Connectedness_and_Health.pd

Chapter Nine References

[1] The Bravewell Collaborative. (n.d.). The Connection Between Mind And Body - The Bravewell Collaborative. Retrieved from http://www.bravewell.org/integrative_medicine/philosophical_foundation/mind_and_body_connection/

[2] Harvard University. (2014, September). How to boost your immune system - Harvard Health. Retrieved from http://www.health.harvard.edu/staying-healthy/how-to-boost-your-immune-system

[3] Rochester University Medical Center. (2011, December). Story - University of Rochester Medical Center. Retrieved from https://www.urmc.rochester.edu/news/story/3370/robert-ader-founder-of-psychoneuroimmunology-dies.aspx

[4] Griffin, M., & Goldberg, J. (n.d.). 10 Stress-Related Health Problems That You Can Fix. Retrieved from http://www.webmd.com/balance/stress-management/features/10-fixable-stress-related-health-problems

[5] Rankin, L. (2011, December). Can Positive Thinking Help You Heal? | Psychology Today. Retrieved from https://www.psychologytoday.com/blog/owning-pink/201112/can-positive-thinking-help-you-heal

[6] Mitchell, M. (2013, March). Dr. Herbert Benson's Relaxation Response | Psychology Today. Retrieved from https://www.psychologytoday.com/blog/heart-and-soul-healing/201303/dr-herbert-benson-s-relaxation-response

[7] Shiffman, R. (2012, January 1). Why People Who Pray Are Healthier Than Those Who Don't | Huffington Post. Retrieved from http://www.huffingtonpost.com/richard-schiffman/why-people-who-pray-are-heathier_b_1197313.html

Made in the USA
Columbia, SC
28 May 2021